The DIABETES Travel Guide

Davida F. Kruger, MSN, RN, CS, CDE

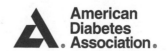
American Diabetes Association®

Director, Book Publishing, John Fedor; *Editor*, Sherrye Landrum; *Production Manager*, Peggy M. Rote; *Composition*, Circle Graphics, Inc.; *Cover Design*, KSA Plus; *Printer*, Transcontinental Printing, Inc.

Printed in Canada
1 3 5 7 9 10 8 6 4 2

The suggestions and information contained in this publication are generally consistent with the *Clinical Practice Recommendations* and other policies of the American Diabetes Association, but they do not represent the policy or position of the Association or any of its boards or committees. Reasonable steps have been taken to ensure the accuracy of the information presented. However, the American Diabetes Association cannot ensure the safety or efficacy of any product or service described in this publication. Individuals are advised to consult a physician or other appropriate health care professional before undertaking any diet or exercise program or taking any medication referred to in this publication. Professionals must use and apply their own professional judgment, experience, and training and should not rely solely on the information contained in this publication before prescribing any diet, exercise, or medication. The American Diabetes Association—its officers, directors, employees, volunteers, and members—assumes no responsibility or liability for personal or other injury, loss, or damage that may result from the suggestions or information in this publication.

⊗ The paper in this publication meets the requirements of the ANSI Standard Z39.48-1992 (permanence of paper).

ADA titles may be purchased for business or promotional use or for special sales. For information, please write to Lee Romano Sequeira, Special Sales & Promotions, at the address below.

American Diabetes Association
1701 North Beauregard Street
Alexandria, Virginia 22311

Library of Congress Cataloging-in-Publication Data

Kruger, Davida F., 1954–
   Diabetes Travel Guide / by Davida F. Kruger.
      p.   cm.
   Includes index.
   ISBN 1-58040-041-8 (pbk. : alk. Paper)
   1. Diabetes—Popular works. 2. Travel—Health aspects—Popular works.
I. Title.

RC660.4 .K784 2000
616.4'62—dc21   00-050219

Dedication

*This book is lovingly dedicated to the two
people who have taught me the most
about diabetes and the importance of
always providing outstanding diabetes care
in every way possible: my mother,
Berenice S. Kruger Levine, and my
mentor, colleague, and friend,
Fred W. Whitehouse, MD.*

Contents

Preface

My mother was diagnosed with diabetes at the age of 30. The 17 years she lived with diabetes were challenging. It was the era before self-monitoring of blood glucose and before we understood the importance of good diabetes control.

In 1982, the year my mother died, I completed my graduate work. I was hired by Fred W. Whitehouse, MD, as a Nurse Practitioner and began my career in diabetes. Through his never-ending support and guidance, I have remained in that position at Henry Ford Health System.

Over the past 18 years, our knowledge of diabetes and of the best care and treatment has changed. However, the disease continues to challenge all who are touched by it. It is my hope that this book will help in some way.

I thank my patients and their families for sharing their knowledge and experiences that added a personal touch and depth to this book. I thank Ann Massirio for her encouragement and review of the manuscript. And I thank my family for allowing me the solitude needed to complete this book and for their ongoing support.

Preparing for Your Trip 1

Whether you're going across the state or around the world, the best approach to travel is to be prepared. And if you have diabetes, that's the *only* way to travel. Plan for as much of the trip as you can. Be curious and ask lots of questions. Questions are the beginning of your "quest" and of being adventurous. Ask questions of health care providers, friends with diabetes who travel, travel agents, and, if you can, people who have been to the location you're going to visit. Try to learn all about the area. Be ready for the unexpected, including cancelled flights, lost luggage, and illness. Do not assume that you will be able to buy your diabetes supplies when you get there. Take what you need and then pack extra. Picture yourself as a prepared and capable traveler, and get ready to have fun!

Do your research

Local libraries and bookstores have many travel books to help you choose and learn more about your destination—climate, terrain, wildlife, culture, foods, and other points of interest. The local library will probably have computers you can use to check the internet and find out more about the places you want to visit. Many states and countries have their own web pages with information about the country and special events as well as lists of places to stay. There are also many websites with information for travelers (see Appendix 1-A). You may have been learning about the place you want to visit for many years, but once you decide to go, start preparing several months in advance.

See your provider early

At least 4–6 weeks before your trip, see your health care provider. You need to schedule this visit far enough in advance so your provider can help you plan. This is a good time to have a physical exam, look at how well your diabetes program is working, make a plan for sick days if you don't already have one, and talk about foot care. This is the time to discuss your travel plans in detail and ask questions that may save you a lot of frustration (or worse) later.

Ask your health care provider to write a letter for you stating that you have diabetes. Also get extra prescriptions for your diabetes medications and supplies that you can carry with you. The letter from your provider should state that you have diabetes and describe your insulin or oral medication program, the adjustments to make for sick days, and if possible, list the phone number of health care facilities or providers in the area you will be traveling through. You should make several photocopies of this letter to take with you, and **always** carry one on you.

For help when you get there

Before traveling you can call ahead to the visitors' bureau of the state or country for help in locating these facilities. Your health care providers may be able to provide you with the name and phone number of a hospital or clinic and provider in the area you will visit.

In the United States, the American Diabetes Association (ADA) can direct you to health care professionals who participate in recognized diabetes education programs and provider recognition programs. These health providers all follow ADA standards of care. You can call 1-800-DIABETES (1-800-342-2383) for more information and referrals to health care professionals in the areas you will be visiting.

Take your prescriptions with you

In addition to taking your diabetes supplies with you (and packing extra), be sure to take a copy of the prescription for each of your medications in case you need more. Ask your provider to write the prescriptions for the generic brand, especially when you plan to travel out of the country. This will make it easier for you to find the medications, because most medications have different trade names throughout the world.

If possible, call ahead to see whether pharmacies in the state you are traveling to will accept prescriptions from a different state. This is usually not a problem, but checking it out ahead of time may save you time and frustration when you get there.

You need a prescription to purchase oral diabetes medications. With the exception of Humalog insulin, many states do not require that you have a prescription to purchase insulin. You may also purchase blood glucose supplies without a prescription. However, when you purchase insulin or blood glucose supplies without a prescription, your insurance does not cover the cost, and you will have to pay full price for the items rather than just your insurance co-pay.

When you travel to foreign countries, you probably will not be able to get your prescription filled. But, if you have the prescription with the generic name of your medication on it, it will be much easier for another physician to help you get the correct medication.

Bring a letter from your doctor

Get a letter from your health provider stating that you have diabetes and you must have your diabetes supplies with you (see Appendix 1-B). This letter comes in very handy, for example, if you have to explain to customs officials why you are carrying syringes, or if you are observing a debate from the seats overlooking the Senate floor in Washington, DC, take out your meter to check your blood sugar, and are abruptly removed from the area by guards who do not know what your meter is.

You should also carry a prescription or letter with information about the insulin and syringes or oral diabetes medications you use (Appendix 1-C). The second letter should state (and you should know) the types of insulin, the concentration (U-100), the dose(s), and the size of your insulin syringe (see

Tables 3-1 and 3-2 on pages 42–46). For diabetes pills, the letter should state the type(s) of pills (see Table 4-1 on page 78), how often to take them, how much to take, and whether they can cause you to have low blood sugar.

Always wear a form of medical identification (Appendix 1-D).

Health insurance know-how

Whether you are traveling out of the state or out of the country, know how your health insurance works. Many health insurance companies will cover the cost of health care throughout the United States. Some companies will only pay for emergency health care in the United States, but you must call a toll-free phone number at the time of care or shortly after for approval. If you are traveling out of the country, it is important to know whether your health care insurance will cover emergency health care. Medicare will not cover health care outside of the United States. If you need coverage, you may contact a travel agent to learn about supplemental health care insurance for the time you are on your trip. Some companies also provide insurance for lost baggage and other things that might disrupt your trip.

Vaccines to keep you healthy

If you are traveling out of the country, find out if you need vaccines or booster shots. Some vaccines have to be given in a series over several weeks or months, so begin early enough to complete the series. Be sure your tetanus booster is up to date.

Then if you get an injury while traveling, it will be one less thing you need to be concerned about. The Centers for Disease Control and Prevention (CDC) can provide you with a list of the vaccines that travelers need. Call the CDC hotline at 1-404-332-4555 or use their website at www.cdc.gov to check which shots you may need for the locations you want to visit. Or you can call a local hospital and ask for their Department of Health Travel or Infectious Diseases. People in these departments can tell you what vaccines you need. Always take a record of your booster shots and vaccines with you when you travel—another of your important papers!

Passports and visas

A passport is an official document stating that you are a citizen of a certain country. It is necessary to have one if you plan to travel outside the United States. In addition to a passport, some countries also require that you get a visa before you go. Obtaining a passport and a visa takes time, so once you know you will be traveling outside the country, start the paperwork. It's worth the effort to get the application into the mail at least 6–8 weeks ahead of time, because it is much easier to obtain these documents through the mail.

How to get a passport

To obtain or renew your passport in the United States, contact your local post office or Clerk of the Court Office for an application. (You may also obtain an application from the website www.travel.state.gov. If you do not have access to the internet, you may be able to use a computer at the public library.) Along with the application, you will need to submit proof of your U.S. citizenship—usually a birth certificate—valid identification, and two identical passport photos of you. The application will tell you where to submit the application.

You may use the National Passport Information center to assist you in applying for a passport. Call 1-900-225-5674, Monday through Friday, 8:30 AM–5:00 PM Eastern Standard Time. The center can answer questions such as where to apply, how to apply, how to complete the application, the status of your application, and other questions you might have. The cost for this service if you use the automated phone line is $0.35 per minute. If you use an operator, the cost for this service is $1.05 per minute. If you have a major credit card, you may call 1-888-362-8668 for the same service at a flat rate of $4.95 per call.

The cost of a passport for new applicants is $60 for those more than 16 years of age and $40 for those under 16. The cost for renewing a passport is $40, and you send in your old one. If you need your passport in less than 25 calendar days, call Passport Services at 1-202-647-0518. (Information is provided in both English and Spanish.) They will assist you in obtaining your passport. In addition to the other requirements, you will need to send a photocopy of your paid round-trip airplane or boat tickets to show the reason you need the expedited services. Your passport can be sent to you as quickly as 3 business days after the application arrives in the Passport Services office. There is a $35.00 fee for express service.

What's a visa?

A visa is a stamp of official approval from a foreign government that is put in your passport. A visa shows that you are allowed to enter the foreign country, your papers are in order, and the purpose of your trip has been approved. Check with your travel agent, the airlines, or the embassy of the country you will be visiting to find out whether you need a visa (see Appendix 8-A). European countries do not require visas.

Website Information

Airline websites: www.airlines.com

Or try www.name of airline.com

Diabetes products: www.Diabetes.WebSite.com

General information: www.diabetes.org

Health care providers: www.tripprep.com

Information on foreign countries:
www.tripprep.com
   A wealth of information for destinations around the world. Includes information on hotels, transportation, currency, diplomatic offices, and safety information.

International Society of Travel Medicine:
Bcbistm@aol.com
   Provides in-depth health and safety profiles of countries around the world. Publishes a list of health care providers in foreign cities. It does not rate or endorse any provider.

Legal travel aid: www.nolo.com

Necessary vaccines information: www.cdc.gov

Passport information: www.travel.state.gov

Travel Health Information: www.travelhealth.com
   Discusses water purity, travel illness, treatments, traveling with medications, and pre-travel checklists.

Travel information around the world:
www.lonelyplanet.com

Travel insurance:
www.aea.com

Insurance information for overseas travel including paying for your trip home if you become ill.

United States Department of State:
www.state.gov

It identifies safety issues and areas of crime and political or civil unrest around the world.

Example of Diabetes Letter

Date:

To Whom It May Concern:

RE: (*Your Name*)

Mr. _____ has diabetes mellitus. As part of his diabetes regimen, it is necessary for him to take insulin and monitor his blood glucose daily. When traveling he must carry insulin, insulin syringes, a blood glucose meter, and lancets

If you have any questions regarding his diabetes care or the supplies he carries with him, please feel free to contact me.

Sincerely yours,

(*Provider's signature*)
Health care provider name _____

Address _____

Telephone numbers _____

_____

Example of Prescription Letter

Date:

To Whom It May Concern:

RE: (*Your Name*)

Mrs. _____ has diabetes mellitus. Her present insulin program requires her to take two injections of insulin daily. Her breakfast dose of insulin is 42 units of NPH human insulin and 18 units of lispro. Before dinner she takes 46 units of NPH human insulin and 22 units of lispro. The insulin is U-100. She uses a 1-cc, 29-gauge, 1/2" insulin syringe.

If you have any questions regarding her diabetes care or insulin dose, please feel free to contact me.

Sincerely,

(*Provider's signature*)
Health care provider name _____

Address _____

Telephone numbers _____

Medical Identification Products

Manufacturer	Product	Features
Apothecary Products 1-800-328-2742 pillminder@aol.com	Necklaces Bracelets Leather key chains	Plastic wallet card with stainless steel medical ID bracelet or necklace, custom-engraved stainless steel or 14K gold necklace or bracelet, and leather key chain with silver-colored medical ID tag.
Goldware Medical 1-800-669-7311 www.medical-id.net	Pendants Bracelets Charms	Fine jewelry in 14K gold and sterling silver, with medical insignia on the front. The back is engraved with your information.
I.D. Technology, Inc. 1-410-602-1911 www.id-technology. com	MediBand Neck chains/ tags Tennis shoe tags Key rings	Distinctively de-signed, low physical–profile watch band accessory is a com-fortable, durable, and discreet emer-gency medical ID.
Identi-Find 1-828-648-6768 www.identfind.com	Iron-on clothing labels	Permanent iron-on labels with your information (4 lines, 30 letters per line).

Manufacturer	Product	Features
	Large-print iron-on name tags Wallet cards	(17 letters/spaces) Folds into 5 sections listing more than 70 items and "authorization for medical treatment" if unable to communicate; vinyl case.
Mcard Corporation 1-708-535-7214	Plastic wallet card Pendant	Computerized medical record containing identification seal, comprehensive medical history, emergency contacts, medications. Free record updates. Free pendant.
Medic Alert 1-800-825-3785 www.medicalert.org	Body-worn emblems Wallet cards	Computerized medical file containing critical medical facts, family and physician contacts. 24-hour phone line with translation of 140 languages. Bracelets and pendants custom engraved with medical facts, personal ID number, and call-collect phone number of the 24-hour line.

Manufacturer	Product	Features
		Gold and silver jewelry, titanium-coated hypo-allergenic, stretch band emblems.
MediCheck International Foundation, Inc. 1-847-299-0620	Neck tags Bracelets Wallet cards	Engraved stainless steel (wallet cards are aluminum); list name, address, phone number, medical condition, medications, doctor's name.
Medicool, Inc. 1-800-433-2469 www.medicool.com	Medicool ID Bracelets Pendants	Engraved medical identification jewelry handmade in California. Bracelets and pendants are sterling silver, gold filled, and 14K and 18K gold.
Miss Brooke's Company 1-888-417-7591 www.Missbrooke.com	Pendants Necklaces	Medical ID pendants with medical caduceus in red. Back of pendant custom engraved with condition, names, phone numbers. Sterling silver or gold vermeil.

Manufacturer	Product	Features
Monroe Specialty Company 1-800-628-0165	Bracelets Necklaces Metal wallet cards	Custom-engraved stainless steel; holds up to six lines; engraved information is colored in red; engraved aluminum wallet card.
Optic Identification 1-888-777-1213 www.idscopes.com	MedScope Pendants Charms	ID pendant attaches to necklace or bracelet. 25 lines of information microfilmed into a magnifier scope. Instant access to emergency information including permission to treat. Plastic, chrome, gold and silver plating.
Scorpio Concepts 1-906-297-6506	Pendants Bracelets	Hand-crafted fine jewelry made of yellow gold, medical insignia in white gold; all 14K.

Manufacturer	Product	Features
SOS America, Inc. 1-800-999-1264 www.sosamerica.com	Bracelets Pendants Watch and sneaker tags	Medical ID jewelry does not require engraving. AMA medical and SOS symbols on two stainless steel halves forming a fire/waterproof capsule protecting 12" non-soluble paper with current medical facts.

From *The Diabetes Forecast Resource Guide 2000.*

Packing for Your Trip 2

Packing the correct items (the ones you'll need) for your trip depends on where you will be going and what you will be doing. The climate and your activities will determine what type of clothes to bring. In addition to clothing, of course, you will pack your diabetes supplies, snacks, and items for an emergency.

If you think through your trip and plan what you may need ahead of time, it always pays off in the long run. You can write down as much of your schedule as you know for each day of your trip and then match your clothing to the schedule. At the same time, you should write down any other items that come to mind so you won't forget to bring them. A checklist is a great help. You can keep the lists that work well and use them for future trips.

Which suitcase?

It is wise to pick the right suitcase for the trip ahead of time. If you will be taking dress clothes, a duffel bag may not be the best protection for your clothing.

You may prefer to use a garment bag that allows you to hang up suits or dresses. If you are traveling to an area where you will be wearing shorts, T-shirts, and a bathing suit, a duffel bag might be just perfect. You may want a suitcase with wheels. Although wheels make a suitcase heavier, rolling a suitcase is easier than trying to carry it. You might fill a nylon duffel bag with your snack foods, and it will have room when it's time to come home for some purchases. A small tote or backpack is usually helpful along the trip and when you arrive at your destination to carry diabetes supplies, snacks, travel papers, maps, camera, and other supplies each day.

Be sure to label each piece of luggage with your name and a phone number. You may want to use a business address on your luggage tag rather than your home address. If someone finds your luggage, you may not want that person to show up at your home unannounced. If you have some type of unusual or colorful tag on your luggage, it'll be easier to spot on the baggage carousel.

Packing twice

It is important to pack twice as much diabetes medication and supplies as you think you will need. The extra supplies will come in handy if you become ill, some get lost, or other problems arise. Never pack your diabetes supplies in the luggage that you are going to check. Keep all diabetes supplies and medications **with you at all times**. If your luggage does not arrive with you, you may need to buy a toothbrush and some new clothes, but you will have your diabetes supplies and medications. If you are traveling with a companion, pack half of your supplies in that person's carry-on bags just in case something happens to yours. It's wise to make a list of the things that belong in your Diabetes Survival Kit (see pages 50–53 and 83–84) to be sure you remember to bring everything you need.

Packing food

Be sure to pack supplies to treat low blood glucose and plenty of healthy snack foods. These are as important as your medications. Travel may be delayed. Airlines have limited food service on many flights. Food on the road is often not nutritional. Carrying several healthy snacks, such as nutrition bars, fruit, or packets of crackers and cheese, can be a great help along the way (see Table 2-1).

Put snacks in re-sealing plastic bags to keep them fresh. Many snacks can be purchased in single serving sizes but may be more expensive that way. Read the labels to see how much carbohydrate is in one serving of the food. To treat low blood glucose you need 15 g of carbohydrate to begin treating it. In addition to the snacks listed in Table 2-1, consider bringing the following:

- One full meal: sandwich, fruit, drink, and dessert
- Single-serving snacks
- Single-serving cereal
- Jar of peanut butter
- Crackers
- Bread

- Chips
- Canned single-serving fruit cups
- Plastic bowl, plastic utensils

At the restaurant where you have dinner, ask for a take-out glass of milk. You can keep it cool on ice or in the mini-bar refrigerator until bedtime. Use it for a bowl of cereal or as part of the bedtime snack.

If you are flying, you can call ahead to see whether a meal will be served during your flight. If a meal will be served, you may request a special meal when you book your flight or at least 2 days before the flight (see chapter 5).

TABLE 2-1. Travel Snacks to Carry

Snacks	Servings (15 g carbohydrate)
Animal crackers	7
Ginger snaps	3
Gold fish, pretzels	1/2 cup
Graham crackers	3
Gummy bears	6
Vanilla wafers	5
Oyster crackers	26
Popcorn cakes	2
Pretzel sticks	35
Pretzel rods	2 1/2
Saltines	6
Granola bars	1/2
Single serving boxes of cereal	1–2
Cheese and cracker packs	1 1/2
Gold fish, cheese, 1 oz pack	1
Raisins	2 Tbs
Juice boxes 6–8 oz	1 1/2
Gatorade 8 oz	1

Packing your trusty monitor

Pack extra blood glucose monitoring supplies. If you run out or lose them, you'll need to know the name of your blood glucose monitor, the blood glucose test strips to use with it, and the type of battery. Write this information down and put it with your important travel papers. Also write down the toll-free phone number of the manufacturer of your monitor. Most companies will ship you a new meter wherever you are if yours malfunctions while it is still under warranty. Whenever possible take a second blood glucose meter with you to use as a backup.

Your insurance company will not purchase a second meter for you, however, so ask your health care providers or pharmacist about special rebate programs. Many companies have rebate programs that will allow you to purchase a second meter at a relatively low cost. You might also want to ask your health care providers whether they have a loaner program. Clinics often have a supply of meters that may be loaned for a short period of time. You will be responsible for keeping the "loaner" meter in good condition.

What else do you put in your carry-on bag?

A carry-on bag that you keep with you at all times makes sense whether you are flying, driving, or traveling by boat or train. You should **always** keep all of your diabetes medications, supplies, and snacks with you. If the bags you check do not make it to your destination, you will still be able to take care of your diabetes. If you have room in the carry-on bag, you may wish to pack clothing for one day, along with books or magazines to read while you travel.

Traveling can make you dehydrated. A bottle of water, lip balm, and hand cream can help make you feel more comfortable. Glasses and contact lens supplies should be kept with you. Travel papers, passports, and maps also belong in your carry-on bag.

Any item you find useful while traveling or that you would be lost without should be in your carry-on bag. It's wise to keep a light sweater or jacket with you when you travel in case it gets cool.

For the sun

If you will be spending time in the sun, whether on a beach, hiking, or skiing, pack sunscreen. Test the sunscreen before you travel to be sure it will not cause a skin rash or irritation. Eye protection from the sun's rays is also important. Be sure to pack sunglasses or ski goggles.

Some medications can cause problems for you if you are in the sun, and it is difficult to predict when sensitivity to the sun will occur. You should use a sunscreen that blocks UV rays if you are taking any medications that can cause you to be sensitive to light (photosensitivity). Your health care provider or pharmacist can advise you about which of your medications can cause a reaction to the sun and tell you when you should try to stay out of the sun (see Appendix 2-A).

Bring your own first aid kit

Put together a first aid kit for traveling. Be prepared for small emergencies or illnesses with the medications that you might need. If you are going out of the country, take items that will help you if you get one of the common traveler's illnesses. The items on the following list are good to have with you.

FIRST AID KIT

☐ Bandage tape 1"

☐ Band-aids

☐ Gauze pads (4" × 4")

☐ ABD pads (2 large gauze pads)

☐ Roll of gauze (Kling)

☐ Ace bandages 2" and 3"

☐ Butterfly tapes (work like stitches to hold a cut together)

☐ Tongue depressors (good splints)

☐ Analgesics (aspirin or acetaminophen)

☐ Thermometer

☐ Sunscreen

☐ Nasal decongestant

☐ Nose spray

☐ Tweezers

☐ Fingernail clipper

☐ Toenail clipper

FIRST AID KIT

(Continued)

☐ Foil-wrapped sterile wipes

☐ Antibiotic cream

☐ Antiseptic (alcohol or betadine)

☐ Cold pack

☐ Scissors

☐ Insect repellent

☐ Calamine lotion (for insect bites, poison ivy, and sunburn)

☐ Motion sickness pills

☐ Injectable glucagon kit (if you take insulin or a diabetes pill that can cause hypoglycemia)

☐ Pepto Bismol

☐ Immodium (for diarrhea)

☐ Sugar-free cough syrup

☐ Antibiotics: Cipro (for diarrhea), Bactrim (for UTI), Z-Pack (for upper respiratory infection) or Levaquin (for UTIs, skin infection, and severe traveler's diarrhea), Keflex (for insulin pump site infection).

☐ Contraceptives

☐ Diamox (for altitude headaches) prescription

☐ Famvir (pills for cold sores)

☐ Tigan suppositories (for nausea and vomiting)

☐ Sanitary products

☐ Bee sting kit

☐ Snake bite kit

Other things to consider packing

You don't need to pack an entire sewing kit, but a few items to get you through in a pinch are helpful: thread in light and dark colors, a needle, a few straight pins, a few safety pins, and several buttons. Some larger hotels provide a small sewing kit for their guests.

Other items you might consider packing include a hair dryer, an iron, or a small hot water pot. To save yourself from having to carry these appliances with you, you could call ahead to see what is provided at the place you will be staying. Most hotels provide all of these appliances at no extra charge. Many hotels have coffeepots in the rooms, which you can use to boil water for drinks, dried soups, or snacks. If you are going overseas, you may need to take plug adapters and a transformer, so you can plug your appliances into the direct electric current used there. Your trip will go more smoothly if you do a little homework before you go, so you know what to expect when you get there.

Which shoes and socks should you pack?

People with diabetes must take very good care of their feet. The best way to do this at home or on a trip is to wear comfortable, well-made shoes that support your feet, such as running or walking shoes of leather or a breathable material. On a trip you should take several pairs of shoes, so that you can change them during the day and prevent blisters from developing.

Neuropathy is a long-term complication of diabetes. It is damage to nerves, most often in the feet. In addition, many people with diabetes also have cardiovascular or heart changes that may interfere with the flow of blood to the feet. In the early stages of neuropathy, your feet may be painful, and this pain may get worse over time. Often the pain is most noticeable during the night. As neuropathy progresses, the pain may go away, but it is replaced with a numbness or lack of feeling. When the numbness occurs, there may be little sensation in your feet. At this stage you will not be able to feel a sore, cut, or blister on your feet. You should be careful to wear shoes that fit you well with no rips or tears in the lining or nails poking through the sole.

No matter where you travel, your clothing should be comfortable and appropriate for the climate. The most important items of clothing are your shoes and socks. Do not buy new shoes and socks for your trip unless you purchase them 2–3 weeks in advance and have an opportunity to wear them daily to be sure they fit you properly. It is important to remember to wear new shoes for only 2–4 hours a day when you are breaking them in. The shoes you take along should be well broken in and comfortable. They should fit your feet and not cause blisters or calluses.

When you purchase new shoes, be sure there is space the width of your thumb from the end of your longest toe to the end of the shoe. There should be some "give" across the top of the shoe at the widest part of your foot. Your toes should have wiggle room. The heel of the shoe should fit snugly enough, so it does not rub up and down against your heel. It is best if the shoe has an arch support. Look for a shoe with a flexible sole. This will help cushion your foot.

Wear socks that cushion your feet, too. Cushioning in newer socks, such as cotton-acrylic blends, will wick perspiration away from your feet. This is good because perspiration or any moisture on your feet or between your toes may cause your skin to break down, and you could get an infection. However, be sure your socks are not too thick for your shoes and do not have thick seams that press on your toes. You should be able to move your toes inside your shoes with the socks on. If your socks are the correct thickness, your shoes fit comfortably and do not feel too tight. There are many socks designed just for people with diabetes. These socks have no seams to irritate your toes and no elastic to cut or pinch feet, and they are made of breathable fabrics (see Appendix 2-B).

A journey of a thousand miles starts with one step

Inspecting your feet every day will be even more important when you are traveling and sightseeing. Each morning and again in the evening, look at your feet for reddened areas, blisters, cuts, scratches, sores, or any other changes. If you need a mirror to see the bottom of your feet, be sure to pack one. You can use a device called the FootSaver to look at the bottoms of your feet. The FootSaver is a mirror attached to the end of a lightweight aluminum pole with a molded grip. The handle is adjustable, and it swivels and telescopes to make it easier for you to look at all parts of your feet. Be sure to check between your toes. If you need help, don't hesitate to ask a traveling companion, who will certainly be affected, too, if you develop foot problems.

It is important to follow some basic routine that can prevent foot infections and other complications from happening. The following list of suggestions will help you keep your feet healthy at all times, at home and away from home.

1. Inspect your feet every day for blisters, cuts, scratches, or reddened areas. Always check between your toes.

2. Wash your feet daily. Dry carefully, especially between the toes.

3. When you are bathing, avoid extreme temperatures. People who have diabetes may have neuropathy or nerve damage to their feet. You may not be able to determine just how hot the water is. Test the water with your elbow (or a bath thermometer) before bathing. This will prevent you from getting burned.

4. If your feet feel cold at night, wear socks. Do not apply a hot water bottle, electric blanket, or heating pad.

5. Do not walk on hot surfaces such as sandy beaches or on the cement around swimming pools. If you must walk in these areas, be sure to wear shoes with a thick enough sole to protect your feet from getting burned.

6. Do not use cold packs on your foot or ankle unless instructed to do so by your health care provider.

7. Do not walk barefoot anywhere, anytime.

8. Inspect the inside of your shoes daily for foreign objects, nail points, torn lining, and rough areas.

9. Do not soak your feet unless specifically instructed to do so.

10. Apply a thin coat of a moisturizing cream daily after bathing. Do not put cream between your toes.

11. Wear properly fitting socks. Do not wear mended socks. Avoid socks with thick seams. Change socks daily. Do not wear garters or anything tight around your legs or feet.

12. Shoes should be comfortable at the time you buy them. Purchase shoes in the afternoon when feet tend to be the largest. Do not depend on the shoes to stretch to fit you.

13. Do not wear shoes without socks or stockings.

14. Do not wear sandals with thongs between the toes.

15. Cut nails straight across or follow the curve of the nail. If nails are thick or difficult to cut, have a health care provider or podiatrist cut them. Don't risk injuring your foot.

16. Do not smoke. Smoking directly affects the circulation to your legs and feet.

17. Do not treat corns or calluses on your own. Consult a health care provider.

18. Never use any medication on your feet without first discussing it with your health care provider.

19. If any changes occur to your feet, contact your health care provider immediately.

20. For more information and a free foot-care kit entitled, "Feet Can Last A Lifetime," call 1-800-438-5383.

Before you go, be aware of the shape your feet are in

In later stages of neuropathy, the structure or shape of your foot may change. The muscles that support the bones in your feet are affected by neuropathy. They may allow the bones in your feet to move, and so your feet change shape. Your feet are also more prone to injury. You might notice that your toes begin to curl under and you walk on the tips of your toes rather than the bottom surface of your feet. The arch of your foot may become flat or more pronounced. Bunions may form. All of these changes put stress on the surface skin of your feet. The stressed areas are where calluses develop, and those areas are most at risk for foot ulcers. Do see your health care provider to discuss the shape your feet are in if you have calluses or your shoes no longer fit well.

If you have neuropathy and changes in the structure of your feet, talk with your provider about getting therapeutic shoes or inserts. These shoes are specially fitted to your feet so they can protect your feet from developing ulcers. Your health insurance may cover some or all of the cost of these specially made shoes. The newer types of therapeutic shoes are more attractive. Some shoes have a larger toe box so your toes will fit comfortably and your feet are protected. Allow enough time to get these shoes, and wear them for several weeks before traveling to be sure they fit you comfortably (see Appendix 2-C).

Medications that May Cause Sun Sensitivity

☐ Antihistamines

☐ Coal tar products (such as Tegrin and Denorex)

☐ Oral contraceptives and estrogen

☐ Anti-inflammatory drugs (such as ibuprofen and naproxen)

☐ Phenothiazines (tranquilizers such as thorazine)

☐ Sulfa antibiotics (such as Bactrim and Septra)

☐ Thiazide diuretics (such as Dyazide)

☐ Tetracycline antibiotics (such as minocycline)

☐ Tricyclic antidepressants (Elavil is used for painful neuropathy)

This list is not final. Review your medications with your pharmacist or health care provider to determine whether any medications you are taking could cause you to be sensitive to the sun.

Socks for People with Diabetes

☐ Rx Comfort Socks   1-888-522-7625

☐ Therasox   1-800-433-2469

☐ Promed European
     Comfort Sock   1-800-433-2469

☐ CareSock Plus   1-800-433-2469

☐ Durasox or Durasox Plus   1-800-433-2469

Medicare's Therapeutic Shoe Bill

For Medicare to pay for your therapeutic shoes, you must have one or more of the following:

a. Neuropathy in your feet and calluses

b. History of calluses leading to ulcers

c. Significant foot deformity

d. Previous amputation of a foot or part of a foot

e. Limited circulation

What types of shoes are covered?

a. Custom-molded shoes

b. Extra-depth shoes

c. Inserts

d. Shoe modifications

Coverage is limited to the following in one calendar year:

a. One pair of custom-molded shoes with inserts and two additional pairs of inserts or,

b. One pair of extra-depth shoes and three pairs of inserts.

c. Modifications of shoes can be substituted for a pair of inserts.

Who provides therapeutic shoes?

Shoes must be fitted and provided by a podiatrist, orthotist, pedorthist, or prosthetist. These professionals must be registered with Medicare. They will fill out the appropriate prescription after your physician has completed the Certification statement.

What is the Certification statement?

The physician who treats your diabetes must certify your need for special shoes.

What are the rules for reimbursement?

The shoe supplier will file the appropriate claim form with Medicare. Reimbursement is limited to 80% of the reasonable charge, and there is a maximum amount that Medicare will reimburse.

Do other insurance companies cover therapeutic shoes?

Many other health insurance companies will also reimburse for therapeutic shoes similar to the way Medicare does. You will need a prescription from your health care provider. Check with your insurance company regarding the coverage they will provide. Your insurance company will also tell you where you can go to be fitted for therapeutic shoes.

Insulin and Your Travels 3

All people with type 1 diabetes take insulin injections. About 40% of people with type 2 diabetes also take insulin. As you well know, it can be tricky trying to time insulin action with the digestion of your meals to keep blood glucose near normal levels. So, following a familiar schedule of meals, snacks, exercise, and injections can help your trip go more smoothly. But so many things can affect your blood glucose level: if you miss a meal or get much more exercise than usual, or you're in a different time zone, or you get ill. And the stress that you feel having to cope with new situations affects your blood glucose, too! So, be flexible and use the information in this book to help you keep your balance.

Being organized is the key to smooth sailing and successful travel. Any change of routine—traveling or staying in a hotel or visiting someone else's home—can make you forget to take your insulin. If you have everything with you in your bag or cooler, you're more likely to remember to use it.

In your carry-on bag

When you pack your insulin, syringes, blood glucose meter, test strips, ketone strips, and glucagon kit, pack twice as many supplies as you think you will need. Keep them with you throughout the trip. Never put them in your checked baggage in case they get lost or damaged en route. Also carry glucose products (Appendix 3-A) and foods to treat low blood sugar and snacks for 24 hours. They might make your tote bag a little heavy at the start of the trip, but they will keep you healthy and relieve you of worry time and again.

If you haven't already, discuss how to use a glucagon kit to treat a serious low blood glucose level with your health care provider (Appendix 3-B). Try to be sure that at least one person traveling with you knows that you have diabetes and how to treat your low blood glucose, including how to use the glucagon if necessary.

One more thing about snacks

If you take insulin, you must have snacks or glucose products with you all the time. You should never risk having low blood glucose anywhere you go. At your destination when you are walking all day sightseeing, you are likely to get more exercise than usual. You'll need an extra snack between meals, preferably protein and carbohydrate, such as cheese and crackers or half a meat sandwich. Children with diabetes need snacks throughout the day and at bedtime, too. On airplanes or at restaurants, they may not like the food available. You might not either. Pack items that you and they will eat to keep on schedule and to prevent low blood glucose. In fact, it will be wise to pack a small suitcase with a variety of snacks. You might start with the list of snacks on page 22.

You can use glucose tablets, gels, or liquid to treat low blood glucose. They are easy to carry, but try them out before you travel. You may not care for the taste or consistency of one of the products.

Your prescription letter

You should also carry with you a prescription or letter from your health care practitioner with information about the insulin and syringes you use (see Appendix 1-C, page 12, for an example of this letter). The letter should state (and you should know) the types of insulin you use, the concentration (Table 3-1), the dose(s), and the size of your insulin syringe (Table 3-2).

Insulin rules of the road

Insulin in opened bottles is safe for about 1 month if you keep it at normal room temperature. It should not get hotter than 86 degrees or colder than 40 degrees. To remember when you opened the bottle, write the date on the label.

When you travel in warm or cold climates, your insulin will need special care. You may choose from a variety of cool packs commercially available to store your insulin at the correct temperature and all your other diabetes supplies, too (see Appendix 3-C). This may be the most important carry-on bag you ever own. Never leave insulin in a car. In warm weather the car will be too warm for the insulin, and in cold weather the car will be too cold. Do not pack insulin

TABLE 3-1. Insulins

Product	Manufacturer	Form	Concentration
Rapid acting (onset 15 minutes)			
Humalog	Lilly	Human	U-100
Humalog cartridges	Lilly	Human	U-100
Short acting (onset 1/2–2 hours)			
Humulin R (Regular)	Lilly	Human	U-100, U-500
Iletin II Regular	Lilly	Pork	U-100
Humulin R cartridges (1.5 ml)	Lilly	Human	U-100
Humulin R Pen (3 ml)	Lilly	Human	U-100
Novolin R	Novo Nordisk	Human	U-100
Novolin R Penfill (1.5 ml and 3.0 ml)	Novo Nordisk	Human	U-100
Purified Pork R	Novo Nordisk	Human	U-100
Novolin BR (velosulin; Regular Buffered)	Novo Nordisk	Human	U-100
Novolin R (Regular)	Novo Nordisk	Human	U-100
Prefilled (1.5 ml)			

Intermediate acting (onset 2–4 hours)

Humulin L (Lente)	Lilly	Human	U-100
Humulin N (NPH)	Lilly	Human	U-100
Iletin II Lente	Lilly	Pork	U-100
Iletin II NPH	Lilly	Pork	U-100
Humulin N Cartridges (1.5 ml)	Lilly	Human	U-100
Humulin N (NPH) Pen (3 ml)	Lilly	Human	U-100
Novolin L (Lente)	Novo Nordisk	Human	U-100
Novolin N (NPH)	Novo Nordisk	Human	U-100
Novolin N Penfill (1.5 ml and 3.0 ml)	Novo Nordisk	Human	U-100
Novolin N Prefilled (1.5 ml)	Novo Nordisk	Human	U-100
Purified Pork Lente	Novo Nordisk	Human	U-100
Purified Pork N (NPH)	Novo Nordisk	Human	U-100

Long acting (onset 4–6 hours)

Humulin U (ultralente)	Lilly	Human	U-100

TABLE 3-1. (Continued)

Product	Manufacturer	Form	Concentration
Mixtures			
Humulin 50/50 (50% NPH, 50% Regular)	Lilly	Human	U-100
Humulin 70/30 (70% NPH, 30% Regular)	Lilly	Human	U-100
Humulin 70/30 Cartridges (1.5 ml)	Lilly	Human	U-100
Humulin 70/30 Pen (3.0 ml) (70% NPH, 30% Regular)	Lilly	Human	U-100
Humalog 75/25 Mix Pen (3.0) (75% NPL [Lispro protamine suspension], 25% Humalog)	Lilly	Human	U-100
Novolin 70/30 (70% NPH, 30% Regular)	Novo Nordisk	Human	U-100
Novolin 70/30 Penfill (70% NPH, 30% Regular; 1.5 ml and 3 ml)	Novo Nordisk	Human	U-100
Novolin 70/30 Prefilled (70% NPH, 30% Regular)	Novo Nordisk	Human	U-100

Insulin Action

Insulin Type	Onset	Peak (hours)	Effective Duration (hours)	Maximum Duration (hours)
Animal				
Regular	0.5–2	3–4	4–6	6–8
NPH	4–6	8–14	16–20	20–24
Lente	4–6	8–14	16–20	20–24
Human				
Lispro	<15 Minutes	0.5–1.5	2–4	4–6
Regular	0.5–1	2–3	3–6	6–10
NPH	2–4	4–10	10–16	4–18
Lente	3–4	4–12	12–18	16–2C
Ultralente	6–10	—	18–20	20–24

TABLE 3-2. Insulin Syringes

Syringe Size (units of insulin)	Insulin Concentration	Needle Gauge (diameter)	Needle Size (length)
1-cc syringes (hold up to 100 units of insulin)			
1-cc	U-100	28G	1/2"
1-cc	U-100	29G	1/2"
1-cc	U-100	30G	5/6"
1/2-cc syringes (hold up to 50 units of insulin)			
1/2-cc	U-100	28G	1/2"
1/2-cc	U-100	29G	1/2"
1/2-cc	U-100	30G	5/6"
3/10-cc syringes (hold up to 30 units of insulin)			
3/10-cc	U-100	28G	1/2"
3/10-cc	U-100	29G	1/2"
3/10-cc	U-100	30G	5/6"

Note: The larger the gauge (30G is larger than 28G), the smaller the diameter of the needle.

in a suitcase that will be checked at an airport. The baggage compartment is not climate controlled.

Some tourist locations, such as amusement parks or water parks that you will be visiting for the day, will often store your insulin in the refrigerator at the first aid station. Call ahead to check before you get to the park. But the best idea is to keep your insulin with you in a protected cool pack.

Make a habit of inspecting your insulin for damage or loss of potency each time you use it. Are there any changes in appearance? Is it discolored? Are there any large particles present in the liquid? Are there salt- or sugar-like crystals gathered on the narrowed portion of the vial? Has your regular or lispro (Humalog) insulin that is supposed to be clear become cloudy? If any of these changes has occurred, the insulin vial should be thrown away. Other changes to the potency are not visible, so be alert for signs that your insulin is not lowering your blood glucose as it should, especially when there is no other explanation. This is true of the insulin for a pump as well. Always date your insulin when you open it, store it correctly, and throw it away after 4 weeks or whenever the manufacturer recommends.

Trash is important

When you're on the road, be sure to dispose of your used syringes, pen needles, insulin pump infusion needle and lines, and lancets safely. Carelessly leaving them in trashcans at motels or restaurants can frighten and endanger other people, and it is illegal. You may purchase a personal size–safety disposal box. It is small enough to fit in your carry-on bag or suitcase. At the end of your trip, it can be disposed of at home following the regulations of your area.

For example, you might choose to use a Safe-Clip, which can be purchased in most drug stores. A Safe-Clip is a small device that clips off the needle of your syringe and automatically stores the needle tip. Although the device is very small, it will store up to 2 years of needle tips, and when it is full, you can dispose of the entire device. The rest of the syringe can

HOW TO STORE INSULIN

Manufacturers of insulin recommend that you store it in the refrigerator. This is to protect it from extreme changes in temperature, which can affect its potency. However, injecting cold insulin can make injections uncomfortable. It is also difficult to keep insulin in a refrigerator when you're on the road. Insulin can be kept at room temperature for 30 days.

The guidelines for storing prefilled insulin pens and insulin cartridges are different. Regular and lispro (Humalog) prefilled pens and cartridges can be used at room temperature for up to 30 days after first use. Prefilled pens containing NPH and 70/30 can be stored at room temperature for 7 days after first use. Pens with 75/25 can be stored 10 days. Keeping your insulin in a cooler or cool pack can protect it from temperature extremes and from being knocked around in a purse or backpack.

be disposed of in the regular trash. This device would save you from having to carry around the syringes until you could safely dispose of them.

You can reuse your insulin syringes, pen needles, and lancets (see Appendix 3-D). Even if you choose not to reuse them when you are home, you may want to reuse them when you travel to cut down on how much you have to carry with you.

Packing your trusty monitor

Pack extra blood glucose monitoring supplies. If you run out or lose them, you'll need to know the name of your blood glucose monitor, the blood glucose test strips to use with it, and the type of battery. Write this information down and put it with your important travel papers. Also write down the toll-free phone number of the manufacturer of your monitor. Most companies will ship you a new meter wherever you are if yours malfunctions while it is still under warranty. Whenever possible take a second blood glucose meter with you to use as a back up.

Your insurance company will not purchase a second meter for you, however, so ask your health care providers or pharmacist about special rebate programs. Many companies have rebate programs that will allow you to purchase a second meter at a relatively low cost. You might also want to ask your health care providers whether they have a loaner program. Clinics often have a supply of meters that may be loaned for a short period of time. You will be responsible for keeping the "loaner" meter in good working order and buying your own blood glucose strips. If you will be taking a second meter with you, be sure you are familiar with the proper way to use it and that you have the correct test strips.

As an emergency backup, if you are going to a wilderness area or somewhere you could not get a new battery or replacement for your meter, you might want to carry some test strips that can be read by eye. You put the drop of blood on the strip and compare the results to a color chart. This is not as accurate as using a blood glucose meter, but it is better than not having a way to check your blood sugar at all.

Check for ketones

You do need to carry ketone test strips with you. If you get ill or if your blood glucose goes higher than 250 mg/dl, it is very important for you to check your urine for ketones.

Ketones in your urine are a warning sign that your body is burning fat for fuel rather than glucose. This could mean that your diabetes is out of control. If you have ketones in your urine, you may need extra insulin. People who have type 2 diabetes do not usually produce ketones in their urine, but if you have type 2 diabetes and become ill, it's a good idea to check your urine for ketones, too. It's the sign of a serious condition developing. Whether you have type 1 or type 2 diabetes, if you have ketones in your urine, contact a health care provider right away.

Several companies now make a blood glucose meter that uses two types of blood glucose test strips. One test strip is designed to monitor blood for glucose. The second test strip is used to check blood for ketones. You may prefer to use this method of testing to check for ketones.

Diabetes survival kit

Put in your survival kit the things that you want to have with you on your travels. Some of them you may already be carrying with you everytime you go out the door. Use this checklist to help you start creating your own survival kit.

KETONE TESTING

If your blood glucose is 250 mg/dl or higher and it cannot be explained by what you have just eaten, check for ketones in your urine.

Equipment:

☐ Ketone test strip

☐ Cup or clean container for sample, if desired

☐ A watch or other timing device

1. Dip a ketone test strip in a urine sample, or pass it through the stream of urine.

2. Time the test according to the directions on the package.

3. The strip will change colors if ketones are present. Compare the test strip to the color chart on the package.

4. Record the results.

■ Insulin supplies

—insulin, syringes, case to dispose of them

—letter or prescription with dose(s) and types of insulin you use

■ Extra prescriptions for diabetes medications and supplies

■ Note from health care provider about your need for diabetes supplies

- Insulated travel bag for insulin
- Medications
- Glucagon kit (Appendix 3-B)
- Glucose tablets or quick-acting low blood sugar treatment
- Meter, test strips, and battery
- Extra batteries
- Extra meter
- Lancing device
- Extra lancing device
- Written directions on how to take your insulin
- Phone numbers of your health care team
- Medical ID stating that you have diabetes (Appendix 1-D)
- Insulin pens
- Pump supplies
- Urine ketone strips
- Snacks (at least twice as many as you think you need)
- Sick-day insulin program
- Off pump–day program
- Notebook and pen
- Moist towelettes
- Hand cream

Watch out! The insulin and syringes are foreign, too

Insulin. Be aware that the names of insulin may be different in other countries. For example, the 70/30 mixture you use may be called 30/70 there. Read the labels very carefully.

The concentration of insulin in the United States is U-100. This means that you get 100 units of insulin in 1 ml of fluid. In Europe and other countries, the concentration of insulin is usually U-40. This means that you get 40 units of insulin in 1 ml of fluid. If, somehow, you have to use U-40 insulin, be sure you also use a U-40 insulin syringe and not the syringes you brought with you. If your usual dose is 20 units of U-100 insulin, your dose will be the same with U-40 insulin as long as you use a U-40 insulin syringe. You will still take 20 units of insulin.

If you use a U-100 syringe with U-40 insulin and do not adjust the dose, you will be taking less than 1/2 of your usual dose of insulin. You need to take 2 1/2 times as much U-40 insulin to get your proper dose. For example, if you usually take 10 units of U-100 insulin, multiply by 2 1/2 to get your new dose of insulin.

$$10 \text{ units} \times 2.5 = 25 \text{ units of insulin}$$

Syringes. Syringes are available in different sizes. The common insulin syringes hold 30, 50, or 100 units of insulin (Table 3-2). The length and diameter of the needle also varies. If you must use a syringe that is different from your usual one, look to see whether the numbers on the side of the syringe are in 1-unit or 2-unit increments. If the numbers are even numbers (2, 4, 6), then the syringe measures 2 units of insulin. If the numbers are odd numbers (1, 3, 5), then it measures 1-unit increments. You need to know so you can draw up the correct amount of insulin.

Insulin pens. Insulin pens were used overseas long before they were used in the United States. If you are presently using insulin pens, you should not have any difficulty finding supplies if you need them (see Table 3-3).

Crossing time zones

If you are traveling to a different time zone, you will have to make adjustments to the time you take your insulin. It is important to adjust your schedule to the new time zone as quickly as possible.

Adjusting insulin

Usually if the time change is less than 3 hours, taking your insulin based on the new time will be fine. If the time change is 3 hours or more, then you must make some changes in the timing of your insulin to make the transition to the new time zone as smooth as possible. You'll also make adjustments in your insulin program on the way home, as you return to your usual time zone. The following sections about insulin adjustments are suggestions, not rules. Discuss how much to adjust your insulin with your health care provider.

TABLE 3-3. Insulin Pens

Device	Insulin Cartridge Size	Delivery Information
Auto Pen (Owen Mumford)	1.5 ml	Autopen AN 3000 delivers 2–32 units in 1-unit increments, Autopen 3100 delivers 1–16 units in 1-unit increments
B-D Pen (Becton Dickinson)	1.5 ml	1–30 units in 1-unit increments
B-D Pen Mini (Becton Dickinson)	1.5 ml	0.5–15 units in 1/2-unit increments
Disetronic Pen (Disetronic Medical Systems)	Open system	Allows for the use of all types of insulin. Delivers 1–80 units in 1-unit increments
Humalog Pen or Humulin Pen (Eli Lilly)	Prefilled 3.0 ml	Prefilled disposable delivers 1–60 units in 1-unit increments
NovoPen 1.5 or 3.0 (Novo Nordisk)	1.5 ml/3.0 ml	NovoPen 1.5 delivers 1–40 units of insulin in 1-unit increments NovoPen 3.0 delivers 1–70 units of insulin in 1-unit increments
Novolin Prefilled (Novo Nordisk)	Prefilled 1.5 ml Pen	Prefilled disposable delivers 2–58 units in 2-unit increments

TABLE 3-3. Pen Needles (*Continued*)

Manufacturer	Pen Needle
Becton Dickinson	B-D Ultra fine original 29G × 1/2" B-D Ultra fine III 31G × 5/16"
Novo Nordisk	Novofine 30
Owen Mumford	Unifine Pen tips 29G either 1/2" or 5/16"

From *The Diabetes Forecast Resource Guide 2000*

Adjusting insulin for one or two time zone changes

The time change is 1 or 2 hours, and you take one or more insulin injections per day.

On the day of travel, take your insulin based on your home time. Begin using the local time in the morning of the first full day at your destination.

Traveling east

You have a time change of 3 or more hours to the east (travel day shortened), and you take one insulin injection a day. On your travel day, you may take your insulin as you usually do or decrease it by 10–20%. On the first full day at your destination, wake on the local time schedule and take your usual dose of insulin. Continue to take your insulin at the same time each day using the local time.

Adjusting for two or more injections a day

On your travel day, decrease the last daily dose of intermediate- or long-acting insulin by 20%. On the first full day at your destination, wake on the local time schedule and take your usual dose of insulin. Continue to take your insulin based on the local time.

For example:

Home

20 units NPH, 10 units regular before breakfast

10 units regular insulin before lunch

20 units NPH, 10 units regular before dinner

Travel

20 units NPH, 10 units regular before breakfast on home time

10 units regular before lunch taken on home time

16 units NPH, 10 units regular before dinner on home time

Destination

20 units NPH, 10 units regular before breakfast on destination time

10 units regular before lunch on destination time

20 units NPH, 10 units regular before dinner on destination time

Traveling west

You have a time change of 3 or more hours to the west (travel day lengthened). You take one insulin injection a day. On your travel day, take your insulin as you usually do. Since the day will be longer, you may need a second injection of insulin in the early evening. If you take only intermediate-acting insulin at breakfast, you may need a second injection of the same insulin before dinner. The injection time should be based on your home time not your destination time. The dose should be 1/3 of your morning dose.

For example:

Home   60 units NPH at breakfast on home time

Travel   60 units NPH at breakfast

               20 units NPH before dinner on home time

Destination 60 units NPH at breakfast on local time

If your morning injection is a combination of intermediate-acting insulin and short- or rapid-acting insulin, then your second injection should be the same combination. The time of the dose should be before dinner based on your home time not your destination time. The dose should be 1/3 of your morning dose.

For example:

Home   40 units NPH, 20 units Humalog at breakfast on home time

Travel	40 units NPH, 20 units Humalog at breakfast
	12 units NPH, 7 units Humalog before dinner on home time
Destination	40 units NPH, 20 units Humalog on local time

If your morning injection is an insulin mix of 70/30, 75/25, or 50/50, take your morning injection based on your home time. Your second injection should be 1/3 of your breakfast injection taken before dinner based on your home time.

For example:

Home	50 units 70/30 at breakfast on home time
Travel	50 units 70/30 at breakfast
	15 units 70/30 before dinner on home time
Destination	50 units 70/30 at breakfast on local time

Another option would be to take your usual morning injection based on your home time. If you eat an extra meal, take an injection of rapid-acting insulin (Humalog) to cover the carbohydrate content of the meal. As a rule of thumb, 1 unit of Humalog covers 15 g of carbohydrate. (But this varies by individual, so be sure to check your blood glucose to see how you respond to it. If you know it, use your specific carb-counting equivalent.)

For example:

Home   60 units NPH at breakfast on home time

Travel   60 units NPH at breakfast

4 units* Humalog at dinner

Destination 60 units NPH at breakfast on local time

Adjusting for two or more injections a day

On your travel day, take your breakfast insulin as you usually do based on your home time schedule. If you take insulin at lunchtime, take your usual dose based on your home time schedule. Take your usual dinner-time Humalog or regular insulin at your dinner meal. If your last daily injection of intermediate- or long-acting insulin is usually at dinnertime, delay it 3 hours and decrease the dose by 20%.

For example:

Home   20 units NPH, 10 units Humalog before breakfast

20 units NPH, 10 units Humalog before dinner

---

* Dinner is a small dinner roll, salad, rice, green beans, chicken, fruit cup, and two cookies. The roll, rice, fruit cup, and two cookies are each a serving of 15 g of carbohydrate for a total of 4 servings. The meal has 60 g of carbohydrate. (4 servings × 15 g of carbohydrate = 60 g of carbohydrate). If you take 1 unit of Humalog for each serving of 15 g of carbohydrate, then you take 4 units Humalog to cover the carbohydrate content of this meal.

Travel	20 units NPH, 10 units Humalog before breakfast on home time
	10 units Humalog before dinner when it's served
	16 units NPH at 9–10 PM based on destination time
Destination	Wake on destination time and take 20 units NPH
	10 units Humalog before breakfast
	20 units NPH, 10 units Humalog before dinner

This example includes insulin taken before lunch:

Home	20 units NPH, 10 units Humalog before breakfast
	10 units Humalog before lunch
	20 units NPH, 10 units Humalog before dinner
Travel	20 units NPH, 10 units Humalog before breakfast on home time
	10 units Humalog before lunch when it's served
	10 units Humalog before dinner when it's served
	16 units NPH at 9–10 PM based on destination time
Destination	Wake on destination time and take 20 units NPH

> 10 units Humalog before breakfast
>
> 10 units Humalog before lunch
>
> 20 units NPH, 10 units Humalog before dinner

If your last daily injection of intermediate- or long-acting insulin is usually at 9–10 PM, take this injection at the same time you would based on your home time and increase this dose by 10%.

For example:

Home　20 units NPH, 10 units Humalog before breakfast

10 units Humalog before lunch

10 units Humalog before dinner

20 units NPH at 9–10 PM

Travel　20 units NPH, 10 units Humalog before breakfast on home time

10 units Humalog before lunch when it's served

10 units Humalog before dinner when it's served

22 units NPH at 9–10 PM based on home time

Destination　Wake on destination time, 20 units NPH

10 units Humalog before breakfast

10 units Humalog before lunch

10 units Humalog before dinner

20 units NPH at 9–10 PM

When you arrive at your destination, wake on the destination time and take your usual insulin doses based on your destination time schedule. Discuss with your health care professional what to do if an extra meal is served. It is possible that you can cover the carbohydrate content of the meal using 1 unit of Humalog for each 15 g of carbohydrate or one starch, fruit, or milk serving. (Again, this varies by individual.)

Adjusting your pump for time zones

Set the insulin pump clock to the destination time zone at any time during your flight. Set your basal rate to a constant daytime basal rate over the 24 hour schedule for the pump while traveling. Measure your blood glucose several times during the trip. Bolus to cover snacks, meals, and elevated blood glucose levels. When you arrive at your destination, reset your multiple basal rates based on your blood glucose readings and the destination time zone.

Insulin pumps

If you wear an insulin pump, pack extra pump supplies, carry the toll-free phone number of your insulin pump company, and pack an extra vial of intermediate-acting insulin (NPH/lente) just in case. Most insulin pump companies are able to ship an insulin pump to you within 24 hours as long as the pump is under warranty. If the pump is not still under warranty, but your insurance company will purchase a new pump for you, you can usually get a new one in several days with the assistance of your health care provider. (This is why you need to take extra insulin with you to use until you get the new pump.)

The pump manufacturer may agree to ship you a loaner insulin pump within 24 hours while the paperwork is being completed and approval is obtained from your insurance company. If your pump is out of warranty and your insurance company will not pay for a new pump, you may purchase a new or rebuilt insulin pump at your own expense.

Most insulin pumps have a warranty of 4 years. Most insurance companies will purchase a new insulin pump if you need one—every 4–6 years. It is a good idea to know the length and extent of the warranty on your insulin pump. You should also know the benefits your insurance company will provide and how often you can get a new insulin pump.

In the meantime, while the details are being worked out, you will need to take insulin by syringe or insulin pen. Some people prefer to use just lispro (Humalog) or regular insulin in multiple injections until a new pump arrives. Others prefer to use an injection of intermediate-acting insulin at bedtime and then multiple injections of short-acting insulin during the day. If the pump will not arrive for several days, you may wish to take intermediate-acting insulin at breakfast and bedtime and short-acting insulin before each meal. You may already have a plan that you use for the days when you do not wear your pump. If you do not have a plan, be sure to discuss this with your health care team when you visit them before you travel. It is best if you have a plan written down and keep it with your important travel papers.

Taking time off your insulin pump

If you remove your insulin pump for a few hours, check your blood glucose several times to see whether you will need to take any insulin by insulin pen or injection. Often, if you've been physically active, you may not need to. If your blood glucose level rises while you're off your pump, you may calculate how long you have been off the pump, determine how much basal rate of insulin you have missed, and take that amount by insulin syringe or insulin pen.

For example:

You remove your insulin pump from 2 PM until 4:30 PM. Your blood glucose at 4:30 PM is 180 mg/dl. Your usual basal rate from 2 PM until 4:30 PM is 0.8 units per hour. You have not received 2 units of basal insulin while you were off your insulin pump.

2 1/2 hours off your pump
× 0.8 units per hour = 2 units of insulin

Take 2 units of Humalog or regular insulin by syringe or insulin pen, or if you will be hooking up your pump at this time, bolus 2 units of insulin.

Another way to figure out how much insulin you need to take is to allow 1 unit of insulin for each 25 mg/dl you wish to lower your blood glucose. If your blood glucose is 200 mg/dl and you wish to lower your blood glucose to 125 mg/dl, you might take 3 units of regular or Humalog insulin. **But you need to know how quickly you respond to insulin**. Some people only need 1 unit of insulin for every 50 mg/dl they wish to lower their blood glucose. The first time you use this formula, try using 1 unit of insulin for every 50 mg/dl you wish to lower your blood glucose. If this does not get your blood glucose level where you would like it, then try using 1 unit of insulin for every 25 mg/dl you want to lower your blood glucose.

If your insulin pump malfunctions and you will be off your insulin pump for 24 hours or more, you will need to take intermediate-acting insulin (NPH or lente). To determine how much intermediate-acting insulin you need add all your basal doses for 24 hours. Take this number and divide by 2, because you will take half of your basal rate insulin in the form of intermediate-acting insulin before breakfast and half at 10 PM. You will continue to take your usual boluses before each meal using regular insulin or Humalog with a syringe or insulin pen.

For example:

Your basal rates are

Midnight to 3 AM	3.0
3 AM to 6 AM	2.4
6 AM to 10 AM	4.8
10 AM to 9 PM	6.6
9 PM to Midnight	2.4

The total daily basal rate of insulin is 19.2 units per day.

$$19.2 \div 2 = 9.6 \text{ units of insulin}$$

Round 9.6 up to 10, so you know to take 10 units of intermediate-acting insulin before breakfast and 10 units at 10 PM. Your pump breaks down at 5 PM on Monday afternoon. Your new pump will arrive on Wednesday by 2 PM. Monday night at 10 PM you take 10 units of intermediate-acting insulin. Tuesday before breakfast take 10 units of intermediate-acting insulin and your usual dose of regular or Humalog insulin. At lunch and dinner take your usual dose of regular or Humalog. At 10 PM take 10 units of intermediate-acting insulin. Wednesday before breakfast take 10 units of intermediate-acting insulin and your usual dose of regular or Humalog insulin. At lunch take your usual dose of regular or Humalog insulin. When your insulin pump arrives, be sure to program your basal rates before you hook it up to you. Stop taking the intermediate-acting insulin.

The new pump

When a new insulin pump arrives, it may not be the same model you were wearing. There may be differences in the way you operate it. Be sure to review how to use the new pump by calling the pump manufacturer's toll-free phone number. They will help you enter your basal rates, learn the bolus function, and understand the basic workings of the new pump, which should be enough until you are back home and can get more training (see Appendix 3-E for some insulin pump company phone numbers).

Over-the-Counter Products to Treat Low Blood Glucose

Product Name/ Manufacturer	Carbohydrate/ Dose	Calories	Form
B-D Glucose Tablets (Becton Dickinson)	5 g/tablet	19	Orange flavored tablets
Dex4 Glucose Tablets (Can-Am Care)	4 g/tablet	15	Orange, lemon, raspberry, or grape flavored tablets
Glucose Tablets (Paddock Laboratories)	5 g/tablet	20	Lemon flavored tablets
Glucose 45 (Paddock Laboratories)	15 g/dose (3 doses/tube)	60	Lemon flavored gel
Glucose 15 (Paddock Laboratories)	15 g/dose (1 dose/tube)	60	Lemon flavored gel
Insta-Glucose (ICN Pharmaceuticals, Inc.)	24 g/1 dose tube	96	Cherry flavored gel

Monojel Insulin Reaction Gel (Can-Am Care)	10 g/packet	46	Orange flavored gel
ReliOn Glucose Tablets (Wal-Mart Pharmacies)	4 g/tablet	15	Fruit punch, orange, raspberry, or grape flavored
Store brand glucose tablets	4 g/tablet	15	Various flavors

From *The Diabetes Forecast Resource Guide 2000*

Injecting Glucagon

1. A glucagon kit has a syringe filled with diluting fluid and a bottle of powdered glucagon. The person helping you must mix the diluting fluid with the powder before it can be injected. The instructions for mixing and injecting glucagon are included in the kit.

2. Inject glucagon in the same way and in the same parts of the body that people inject insulin. It may also be given into a muscle or in an IV.

3. If glucagon is mixed in a syringe but not used, you may refrigerate the capped syringe and store it for up to 2 days. Contact the manufacturer for more details.

4. The person with low blood glucose should respond to the glucagon injection in 15–30 minutes. If he or she does not respond, call emergency personnel (911 in the U.S.).

5. The person will probably feel nauseated or vomit. Keep him turned to the side.

6. As soon as the person can swallow, offer regular soda, crackers, or toast.

7. Then offer a sandwich or protein snack.

8. Check blood glucose.

Carrying Cases with an Insulin Cool Pack

These cases help you organize your diabetes supplies. They vary in size and will fit specific needs. The ones listed here all have cold gel packs to protect insulin from temperature changes.

☐ Insul-Vial—Apothecary Products

☐ Insulated Diabetic Wallet—Apothecary Products

☐ FRIO Wallets—Frio Cooling Products

☐ Dia-Pak—Medicool, Inc.

☐ Insulin Protector—Medicool, Inc.

☐ ProtectAll Pack—Medicool, Inc.

☐ The Wallet Organizer—Medport

☐ The 3-in-1 Organizer—Medport

☐ The Daily Organizer—Medport

☐ The Travel Organizer—Medport

☐ Insul-totes—Palco Labs

From *The Diabetes Forecast Resource Guide 2000.*

Reusing Syringes

1. Carefully recap the syringe when you aren't using it.

2. Don't let the needle touch anything but clean skin and your insulin bottle stopper. If it touches anything else, don't reuse it.

3. Store the used syringe at room temperature.

4. There will always be a tiny, even invisible, amount of insulin left in the syringe. So use one syringe with just one type of insulin to avoid mixing the insulins. For this reason, reusing syringes in which you have mixed insulins is not recommended.

5. Do not reuse a needle that is bent or dull. However, just because an injection is painful, doesn't mean the needle is dull. You may have hit a nerve ending or have wet alcohol on your skin, if you use alcohol to clean the injection site.

6. Do not wipe your needle with alcohol. This removes some of the coating that makes the needle go more smoothly into your skin.

7. When you're finished with a syringe, dispose of it properly according to the laws in your area. Contact the city or county sanitation department for information.

From *The American Diabetes Association Complete Guide to Diabetes, 2nd Edition.*

Insulin Pump Phone Numbers

Minimed

In the U.S.	800-933-3322
From outside the U.S.	818-368-2588
France	011-33-46-4316-16
Germany	011-49-172629117
Sweden	011-46-4045-4040

Disetronic Medical System

Country	Telephone Number
Argentina	+54 / 11 4951 0875 1 4988 9100
Australia	+61 / 29 417 79 55
Austria	+43 / 1 801 01 2544, 2545
Belgium	+32 / 1 677 89 31
Brazil	+55 / 11 5092 2547
Canada	+1 / 905 814 6350
Czech Republic	+420 / 5 412 408 38
France	+33 / 1 64 73 34 50
Germany	+49 / 6196 50 50 0
Great Britain	+44 2476 531 338
Hong Kong	+852 / 288 75 175
Hungary	+36 / 1 2422146
Israel	+972 / 3 5773800

Country	Telephone Number
Italy	+39 / 035 219 777
Korea	+82 / 2 747 5999
The Netherlands	+31 / 347 37 31 75
New Zealand	+64 / 9 629 0823
Poland	+48 / 22 663 43 39
Saudi Arabia	+966 / 1 465 03 71
Scandinavia	+46 / 8 601 29 00
Finland	+358 / 9 8520 2130
Norway	+47 / 33 05 55 20
Slovakia	+42 / 1 822326539
Spain	+34 / 91 500 34 84
Cataluna	+34 / 93 455 60 23
Switzerland	+41 / 34 427 12 55
Taiwan	+886 / 2 29411899 +886 / 2 29447499
Turkey	+ 90 / 232 425 1961
U.S.	+1 / 612 795 5200
For all other countries	+41 / 34 427 11 11

Diabetes Pills and Your Travels

Organization is the key to smooth sailing and successful travel. Any change of routine, such as traveling or staying in a hotel or someone's home, can make you forget to take your diabetes pills. You might not think that's true, but it happens, even when you are at home and someone or something disrupts your daily routine.

If you don't already have one, it might be a good idea to get one of those plastic pill organizers with sections for the days of the week, so you can tell at a glance whether you have taken your pills. These organizers are lightweight and can be carried with you in your tote bag or backpack for the day. As always, it is very important that you keep your diabetes medications with you at all times.

It's also important to check your blood sugar, especially when you're under stress or getting more physical activity than usual. Both can have a significant effect on your blood glucose levels.

A meal plan is quite important

If you have a meal plan and it works pretty well with your medications and exercise, then it will help you a great deal if you can continue to eat the same number of meals and snacks on your trip that you are accustomed to having. (That's a reason to carry some food with you, so you can eat when you usually do.) Also, the meals and snacks should contain about the same amount of carbohydrate as the meals at home. You may have to be creative to fit local dishes into your meal plan, so ask your dietitian for help with this. Do some research before you go to find the amount of carbohydrate in the foods you will probably find at your destination, because it's carbohydrate that makes blood glucose rise. For instance, one flour tortilla contains 15 g of carbohydrate, just as one slice of bread and 1/3 cup of rice do. To help you with your research, the ADA has several handy books with lists of the nutrients in many foods. You can also find this information in books in the library.

Carry food with you

You never know when you might be unable to find something to eat or you might not like what is available. Or when the tour bus will break down in the middle of the jungle. Or when the schedule of the relatives you're visiting doesn't match your own. You should always have at least one snack with you, such as cheese and crackers, fruit, a nutrition bar, or some boxes of juice. You may be the only person on the plane with something to eat! Check pages 21–22 for more snack ideas.

If your diabetes pills can cause you to have low blood glucose, you need to have food or glucose products (Appendix 3-A) with you to raise your glucose level. Find out from your health care provider if this is a concern for you.

A letter from your provider

As we discussed in chapter 1, it is important to carry with you a letter from your health care provider stating that you have diabetes, and you need to have your diabetes meter and lancets with you (Appendix 1-B, page 11). You also need to bring extra prescriptions for your diabetes pills in case you need to buy more. You should know which pills you are taking (Table 4-1), but also carry a letter listing the diabetes pills, the dosages, and the times you should take them. The letter might also say whether your medication can cause low blood glucose and what to do about it, in case others need to help you.

Can your diabetes pills cause low blood glucose?

You need to know the answer to this question. Diabetes medications work in different ways to balance the effect of the food that you eat (Table 4-2). If your diabetes medications (especially if you take several of them) can cause your blood glucose to go too low, then you need to always carry glucose tablets or snacks with you to treat low blood glucose.

Diabetes medications that can cause low blood sugar are the sulfonylureas, repaglinide (Prandin), and insulin.

TABLE 4-1. Diabetes Oral Medications

Medication Class	Generic Name	Brand Name
Alpha-glucosidase inhibitors	Acarbose Miglitol	Precose Glyset
Biguanides	Metformin	Glucophage
Meglitinides	Repaglinide	Prandin
Sulfonylureas	Glimepiride	Amaryl
	Glipizide*	Glucotrol
	Glyburide*	DiaBeta Glynase Micronase
	Tolbutamide	Orinase
	Tolazamide	Tolinase
	Chlorpropamide	Diabinese
	Acetohexamide	Dymelor
Thiazolidinediones	Pioglitazone	Actos
	Rosiglitazone	Avandia
Insulin	Insulin	Several

The sulfonylureas are:

- Glimepiride (Amaryl)

- Glipizide (Glucotrol)

- Glyburide (DiaBeta, Glynase, Micronase)

- Tolbutamide (Orinase)

- Tolazamide (Tolinase)

- Chlorpropamide (Diabinese)

- Acetonhexamide (Dymelor)

TABLE 4-2. Action of Oral Medications

Medication Class	Site of Action	Action
Alpha-glucosidase inhibitors (e.g., Acarbose, Miglitol)	Digestive system	Slows the breakdown of starches to glucose. Slows the entry of glucose into the bloodstream after a meal.
Biguanides (e.g., Metformin)	Liver, muscle	Decreases glucose production by the liver.
Meglitinides (e.g., Repaglinide)	Pancreas	Stimulates insulin release by the pancreas in response to a meal.
Sulfonylureas (e.g., Glyburide or Glipizide)	Pancreas	Stimulates insulin release by the pancreas.
Thiazolidinediones	Muscle, liver, fat cells	Enhances glucose uptake by the muscle.

Repaglinide (Prandin) should be taken with meals to avoid low blood glucose. If you have to skip the meal, skip the pill, too. The other diabetes pills do not cause low blood glucose when taken by themselves. But, when you take two different pills (or pills and insulin), your risk of having low blood sugar increases.

Watch out for feeling shaky, nervous, and sweaty. These are some of the warning signs from your body that your blood glucose is dropping below normal.

The reason could be taking too much diabetes medication, a skipped meal, extra exercise, a drug interaction between your diabetes medication and another medication you are taking, or a change in the way your kidneys or liver are working. Check your blood glucose and if you are experiencing low blood sugar, you need 10–15 g of quickly absorbed carbohydrate, such as 1/2 cup of milk or orange juice, 2 teaspoonsful of sugar, 5 or 6 Lifesavers, or 3 glucose tablets. Some diabetes pills slow down the absorption of carbohydrate, such as acarbose (Precose) and miglitol (Glyset). For these you will need to use a glucose product instead of food to bring your blood sugar back up. Glucose products come in tablet, gel, and liquid forms (Appendix 3-A, pages 68–69).

What if you forget to take a pill?

As a general rule, you can take a missed dose of any medication as soon as you remember it. But if it is almost time to take the next dose, just take that dose on time. Do not take a double dose. However, the case is different for some diabetes pills that should be taken with meals. If you miss a dose of repaglinide (Prandin), and you take it between meals, you could end up with low blood glucose. So, don't take it between meals. If you miss a dose of acarbose (Precose) or miglitol (Glyset), you should just take the next pill at the next meal, since its job is to slow the absorption of high-starch carbohydrate foods.

Time zone changes

If you take pills to control your diabetes and will be traveling to a time zone 3 hours or more from your own, you may have to change the time you take your medication. Discuss this with your health care provider and write down the instructions so you can take them with you. If you are told to take your pills with meals, ask whether you should take a pill even if you have to skip a meal.

Physical activity

When you are on vacation, your activity level may increase quite a bit, and you may have problems with low blood glucose. You may need to eat an extra snack between meals containing carbohydrate and protein, such as cheese and crackers or half a meat sandwich. Check your blood glucose every 4 hours and be aware that exercise can keep lowering blood glucose into the next day.

You might also wonder whether you can lower the dose of your pills to counteract the effect of the exercise. Except for repaglinide (Prandin), acarbose (Precose), or miglitol (Glyset), making adjustments to your dose does not have an immediate effect on your blood sugar level. It is more difficult to adjust oral meds than it is to lower insulin by a few units. Some diabetes pills may be cut in half. Check with your pharmacist about the pills you take. The problem is that cutting pills in half does not mean that you will get a correct dose, and it may alter the way your body is able to absorb and use the medication.

Most oral diabetes medications do come in a variety of dosages. Ask your health care provider about the smaller-dose pills, and whether you might take them on the days that you are very active. For example, your dose of medication is a 10 mg pill at breakfast and 10 mg pill at dinner. That same medication may come in a 2.5 mg pill or a 5 mg pill. Request a prescription for the 2.5 mg pill. Instead of taking one 10 mg pill before breakfast and one 10 mg pill before dinner, you would take four 2.5 mg pills before breakfast and four 2.5 mg pills before dinner. Then on the days you are active and your blood glucose levels are running low, you could adjust your dosage by taking only three 2.5 mg pills before breakfast and three before dinner. You'll need to check your blood glucose frequently to help you decide whether you need to adjust your medication and how much.

The effects of illness

People who have type 2 diabetes do not usually produce ketones in their urine, but if you have type 2 diabetes and become ill—especially if you have vomiting and diarrhea so that you are dehydrated—check your urine for ketones. It's the sign of a serious condition developing. If you have ketones in your urine, contact a health care provider right away.

Diabetes survival kit

Use this list to create your own survival kit, and you may want to carry it with you everyday.

- Oral diabetes medications
  - Letter giving dosage and directions for when and how to take them
- Letter from health care provider stating your need for diabetes supplies

KETONE TESTING

If you get ill or if your blood glucose goes higher than 250 mg/dl, and it cannot be explained by what you have just eaten, it is very important to check your urine for ketones. Ketones in the urine are a warning sign that your body is burning fat for fuel rather than glucose. This could mean that your diabetes is out of control.

Equipment:

- Ketone test strip
- Cup or clean container for sample, if desired
- A watch or other timing device

1. Dip a ketone test strip in a urine sample, or pass it through the stream of urine.

2. Time the test according to the directions on the package.

3. The strip will change colors if ketones are present. Compare the test strip to the color chart on the package.

4. Record the results.

- Extra prescriptions for diabetes medications and supplies

- Written directions for how and when to adjust your dosage

- Glucagon kit (if your diabetes medication can cause low blood glucose) (Appendix 3-B)

- Glucose tablets or other quick-acting treatment for low blood glucose
- Meter, test strips, and battery
- Extra batteries
- Extra meter
- Lancing device
- Extra lancing device
- Phone numbers of your health care team
- Medical ID on you stating that you have diabetes (Appendix 1-D)
- Urine ketone strips
- Snacks (about twice as many as you think you need)
- Sick-day program
- Moist towelettes
- Hand cream
- Notebook and pen

Travel by Auto, Plane, or Boat 5

Travel by Auto

When you travel by auto, you can be on your own schedule in the comfort of your own car or one you have rented. You don't need to be as concerned about the size and type of suitcases you pack as long as they fit in the car. The number and types of meals and snacks that you can enjoy at a restaurant or rest stop is only limited by your imagination. Although a person with diabetes can certainly travel alone, it is a good idea to have a traveling companion to share the driving, if possible.

Decide ahead of time how long you will drive before you stop to stretch—about every 2 hours is a good plan. Check your blood sugar at the rest stops to be sure it doesn't drop too low while you are driving and increase your risk of having an accident. Keep rapid-acting carbohydrate such as fruit juice boxes or glucose tablets on the seat next to you in case you need them.

To prevent fatigue you need to stop at regular intervals and stretch. Not only does this help your circulation, but it also protects you from the hypnosis-like effect that long drives can cause. Take a cellular phone with you in the car to use for any emergencies that may arise. Keep identification on you and in the car stating that you have diabetes. If you have an accident, you want everyone who comes to your aid to know that you have diabetes.

Contact AAA or another auto club or go online to get detailed maps of the area you will be visiting. These maps can help you navigate to your destination and warn you of any construction or detours along the way. Also pack a general map of the states you will be traveling through. Both you and your traveling companions should be familiar with the maps before you leave. A flashlight and extra batteries will help you read the maps or find items in the car during dusk and night driving without having to turn on the overhead light and disturb the driver.

Your feet and how they travel

When you sit in a car for several hours, your feet swell because body fluids pool in them. That's why it's good to stop every few hours, walk around, and stretch; it helps your circulation and decreases the swelling. If swelling becomes a problem, consider sitting in the rear seat when you are not driving and putting your feet up—higher than your heart if possible. Pack a few pillows to use to elevate your feet.

Even when you are sitting in the car and not walking, it is important to wear comfortable shoes and socks. Shoes with laces may be better because you can loosen them to allow for swelling. Never drive barefooted or in sandals.

Blood glucose levels

For many people sitting in a car on a long trip will raise their blood glucose levels. High blood glucose can make you feel drowsy or irritable and may cause you to have blurred vision. If you already know that sitting in a car for long periods of time causes you to have high blood glucose, you may want to eat fewer carbohydrates at each meal. If you're driving, you must check your blood glucose at least every 2 hours.

If you take insulin and your blood glucose numbers are higher during your trip, you may want to increase your quick-acting insulin (Humalog) or short-acting insulin (regular), depending on which one you take, by 1 or 2 units before meals. Discuss how to do this with your health care provider or diabetes educator. Choose one or the other: either limit your carbs at meals or increase your insulin, but don't do both at the same time or you risk going too low.

Most important of all, you must check for low blood glucose. If you have low blood glucose, you cannot respond quickly to what is happening on the road, and you are at increased risk for having an accident. Do not rely on how you feel. It is important to check your blood glucose at least every 2 hours to know exactly where it is. Be sure to always have snacks, such as juice or raisins and glucose tablets or gel (Appendix 3-A) to treat low blood glucose on the seat within your reach.

What if you get low while driving?

If you think you are having low blood sugar while you are driving, take 15–30 g of carbohydrate, such as

1 or 2 juice boxes or 3 glucose tablets, and immediately find a place to pull off the road. Check your blood glucose. Do not drive until all your symptoms are gone and your blood glucose has returned to normal (higher than 80 mg/dl). If it is time for a meal, take the time to eat. If you have a driving companion, this is the time to change drivers. Keep a cooler with you in the car with meals and snacks in it. Always pack a meal that can be eaten if you cannot find a restaurant, get into a traffic jam, or get lost. Pack twice as much food as you think you'll need. Try to keep your meals on schedule to prevent high blood glucose and low blood glucose.

Taking care of your insulin

If you take insulin, you need to keep it from getting too hot or too cold. Insulin can be kept in the food cooler as long as it is not touching ice, or you may keep it in an insulin cool pack (Appendix 3-C). Keep all insulin with you inside the car, not in the trunk, where it can get too hot or too cold. When you leave your car, take the insulin with you even if it is in the cooler, or you may want to keep it in a little cooler of its own. On the rare occasion that the car is stolen, you will still have your insulin and blood glucose monitoring equipment.

Taking care of your eyes

Wearing sunglasses helps you avoid glare and protects your eyes. If you wear contacts, be sure to bring extra lenses and lens solution with you. It is also a good idea to bring prescription glasses and sunglasses in case you are unable to wear your contact lenses for any reason.

In the trunk

Any items that are kept in the trunk should be things that you can wait to get to at regularly scheduled stops. You can pack bottled water or a container of water that you can refill at rest stops. Freeze the bottles before you leave on the trip. This will keep the water cold during much of the trip. It can also keep other items in a cooler cold. You can also pack other types of fluids in your cooler, such as sugar-free drinks or juice.

CAR TRAVEL CHECKLIST

(For inside the car)

- [ ] Blood glucose monitoring supplies
- [ ] Insulin and supplies
- [ ] Insulin cool pack
- [ ] Cooler
- [ ] Snacks
- [ ] Meal in cooler
- [ ] Glucose tablets or other quick-acting glucose
- [ ] Bottles of water
- [ ] Other fluids such as sugar-free soda and juice
- [ ] Sunglasses
- [ ] Cellular phone
- [ ] Maps
- [ ] Flashlight and batteries
- [ ] Medic alert ID in car and on person
- [ ] Comfortable shoes and socks
- [ ] Pillow
- [ ] Blanket
- [ ] Sweater or light jacket

Travel by Plane

Traveling by airplane is usually the quickest way to get to your destination. Most flights are on time, but you should be prepared for delayed or cancelled flights and lost baggage. Carry all your diabetes supplies and important papers. Also bring all the food that you might need with you. Airlines prefer not to provide meals. Often you are only given a drink and a bag of pretzels. The contents of your carry-on bag (see chapter 2) will help make your trip go smoothly.

When you make your reservations, ask if a meal will be served. You may request a special meal for people with diabetes at that time or within 48 hours of departure. Most special meals include a good variety of vegetables and fruit and only limited desserts. When you call the airline or your travel agent to request a special meal, ask what is on the menu. You know best what your dietary needs are. In some instances, the meal that is to be served to all the passengers may suit your needs, too.

When booking your flights, try to get a direct flight. If you must take a flight with a connection, look at the in-flight airline magazine for the map of the airport where you have to change planes. This can help you find the gate for your next flight more quickly. If the distance is manageable, the walk will provide you with some exercise after sitting for a long time.

If you are concerned that the distance between the two gates or to the baggage claim area is greater than you are able to walk, request wheel chair or motor cart assistance. You can do this ahead of time over the phone or when you check in. The flight attendant can also request a wheel chair or motor cart to get you to your gate prior to the plane landing. An airline representative will meet you and take you to your connecting gate. The airline is happy to help you with this, so don't let embarrassment keep you from taking good care of yourself.

Where do you want to sit?

Request a bulkhead or emergency exit aisle seat. These seats have maximum legroom, and it will be easier for you to get up and move around periodically. An aisle seat on any row would be the next best choice. On longer flights take the opportunity to get out of your seat and stretch. When the aisles are clear, walk up and down to keep your circulation moving and decrease swelling in your feet. Be sure to wear comfortable shoes that you can wear socks with. Often flights are cool and socks will keep your feet warm. You can always carry another pair of shoes to change into at your destination if you are going to a warm climate.

When you board the airplane, take a pillow and blanket from the overhead compartments. There are not enough for all passengers, so it's first come first served. You might want to cover your legs and feet with the blanket and use the pillow to nap. On long flights, folding the blanket and using it to elevate your legs will help with circulation and decrease swelling in your feet.

Dry as a desert

The air inside the airplane is dry. Carry a bottle of water to drink while you fly. The flight attendant can refill it for you or you can refill it in the rest room. Drink plenty of non-sweetened fluids. Avoid alcohol and limit caffeine. This will help prevent dehydration. Carry lip balm and hand cream and apply them during the flight.

Onboard diabetes care

Carry food and snacks with you to get you through the flight and prevent low blood glucose. Remember that when you are inactive, such as sitting on an airplane, your blood glucose may be higher than usual. It is important to check your blood glucose on a regular basis while you're flying.

Most airplane restrooms have a section of the wall designed for you to dispose of your insulin syringes and lancets safely. You may also choose to put your used equipment back in your carry-on bag to dispose of them when you reach your destination. Do not dispose of them in the regular trash or on your meal tray.

What if you cannot go?

Each airline has their own policy regarding flight changes or cancellations if you become ill prior to traveling or while you are traveling. Be sure to ask the airline or your travel agent for the policy of the airline you will be using. Get the policy in writing. Also get the names of contact people and phone numbers at the airlines that are available 24 hours a day in case you need assistance in changing your flights because you are ill. You can also ask your travel agent about getting trip insurance, which will reimburse you for trips or tours that you had to cancel and the airlines or the tour company would not cover.

Frequent flyers

If you are a frequent flyer or have access to points or coupons to upgrade to first class, this will be helpful on longer flights. First-class seats are larger and provide more legroom. Often the seat works like a recliner chair and the leg rest can elevate your feet. Meal service is more frequent and more predictable because there are fewer passengers to serve and the food is of a higher quality.

A helping hand

If you will be bringing your own wheel chair, walker, or cane, the airlines will make arrangements to help you to your seat and store your equipment. When your flight lands, your equipment will be returned to you, and you will be assisted off the flight. Let the airlines know when you make your flight arrangements of any special needs you have. When you check in, tell them again that you will need special assistance. You will find that you are given first-class treatment in these situations, so don't be hesitant about it at all.

Air sick?

Take medication such as Dramamine (pills) or Scopolamine (patches) with you to prevent motion sickness. It is best to take (or apply) them 30 minutes before you fly. These medications will usually make you drowsy.

More about luggage

Most luggage arrives at your destination without delay; however, if your bag does not appear on the carousel after all the luggage has been unloaded, go to the airline office located in the baggage claim area and report your missing luggage. The airline will want to know exactly what your bag looked like, what you have in it, and how it was labeled. Always put an identification tag on your luggage. It is also a good idea to label the inside of your luggage, too, just in case your luggage tag comes off. Most delays are caused because your luggage did not get on your flight either at the beginning or on the switch to a connecting flight. Usually your luggage will arrive on the next scheduled flight. While this may cause you some inconvenience, if you have packed your carry-on bag carefully, you will have enough supplies to get you through until your luggage arrives.

When your luggage arrives at the airport, the airline will deliver it to you. If your luggage is lost and not recovered, you can make a claim to the airlines to replace what you have lost. On domestic flights, federal regulations limit the amount an airline must pay you to $250 for your lost or damaged luggage and its contents. If the contents of your luggage is worth more, then you may declare this at check in, up to the airlines maximum coverage, which usually is between $250 and $500. The airline will ask you to pay an additional fee to obtain this extra coverage. You might consider flight insurance or trip insurance to cover your luggage depending on the value of its contents. Be sure to pack jewelry and other valuable items in your carry-on baggage.

On international flights, coverage for missing or damaged luggage is covered by the Warsaw Convention. Damages are calculated based on the weight of your luggage. The value of your lost luggage is reimbursed at the rate of $9.07 per pound. If your luggage was not weighed prior to departing, then the airline will assume that all your luggage weighed 70 pounds, and you will be reimbursed $634.90. There are time limits for when you may make a claim, so check your luggage for missing or damaged goods, and report it immediately to the airline.

Travel by Boat

Cruises

Most cruises usually combine airline travel with sea travel in order for you to get to your port of departure. Most cruises are sold in packages that include your air travel. When you choose your cruise, you will have the opportunity to pick your cabin. You will need to decide what type of bed you want and on which deck you want your cabin. Most cruise lines have pictures with descriptions and diagrams of the ship. Ask to see the diagram to help you make your decision. If you have a tendency for seasickness, you might prefer a cabin that is well above the water level. If you have trouble walking or have any handicap that will make it difficult to get around, you should choose a cabin near the dining rooms. Work with your travel agent or the cruise line to pick the cabin that will best suit your special needs.

Menus for meals are prepared before departure. Most cruise lines offer many choices at each meal, and there are opportunities to eat more than three

AIRPLANE TRAVEL CHECKLIST

(Carry-on bag)

- ☐ Airline tickets
- ☐ Passport
- ☐ Hotel reservation information
- ☐ Car rental information
- ☐ Other important papers
- ☐ Jewelry or other valuables
- ☐ Blood glucose monitoring supplies
- ☐ Insulin and supplies
- ☐ Insulin cool pack
- ☐ All medications
- ☐ Snacks
- ☐ Bottle of water
- ☐ Glucose tablets or other quick-acting glucose
- ☐ Map of airport you are connecting through
- ☐ Medic Alert in your tote and one on your person
- ☐ Comfortable shoes and socks
- ☐ Sweater or lightweight jacket
- ☐ Lip balm
- ☐ Hand cream
- ☐ Dramamine (pills) or Scopolamine (patches) for air sickness

meals per day. Passengers are assigned a seating time for dinner, but other meals usually have a range of times you can eat. Your travel agent or the cruise line can provide you with a list of meal times and menus that you can review before traveling. If your diabetes program requires you to eat at a specific time each day, be sure to request the meal times when you choose your cruise and request a specific seating for dinner. Although the meals on a cruise offer you a great deal of variety, you may request special meals at this time as well.

Check ahead of time to see if your cabin will have a small refrigerator to store your insulin. If you do not have a refrigerator in your cabin, your extra insulin can be stored in the refrigerator of the medical clinic on the ship. Keep the insulin you are using in an insulin cool pack (Appendix 3-B). The cool pack inserts can be frozen in the refrigerator of the medical facility.

What if you become ill?

Ask specifically about the cruise line's cancellation policy or reimbursement policy if you are ill prior to the trip and are unable to travel. Also, ask about their policy if you become ill during the trip and must leave the trip early. Obtain the policy in writing. Ask for phone numbers and names of individuals you can contact directly. Most cruise line policies are fairly rigid. You want to be sure you understand the policies of the cruise line before you put down a deposit.

Determine what arrangements can be made to fly you home from one of the ports of call if you are ill. You may need to purchase special trip insurance to protect yourself. You may also wish to obtain a credit card that covers illness and special or medical care of the owner while traveling. For example, the Platinum American Express card or a Gold MasterCard generally covers these costs and the costs of having you airlifted home. Call your credit card company to see what travel benefits you may have.

Settling in

When you have settled into your cabin, introduce yourself to the health care team in the ship's medical facility. Most ships have a physician and nursing staff on board for the duration of the trip. They can be helpful if you become ill on the trip.

Be sure to keep snacks or a form of glucose in your cabin to treat low blood sugars or if you need food before you go to sleep. Food is readily available during the day for mid-morning or afternoon snacks if needed. Always carry a form of glucose with you in case you need to treat low blood sugar. (Appendix 3-A). The ship is big, so do not count on being able to get back to your room to treat low blood sugar.

Let's get physical

Pack comfortable clothes and shoes. There will be plenty of opportunities to get exercise on the ship. In addition to using the indoor health club, you may walk around the decks. Most ships also have swimming pools you can use.

In the sun

Remember that the sun can be stronger when it reflects off the water. Use sunscreen, sunglasses, and a sun hat. You might want to wear lightweight long-sleeve clothing for part of the day to protect yourself from overexposure to the sun. Be aware that sunbathing may cause low blood sugar.

Motion sickness?

Be sure to carry medication for motion sickness. You may wish to take this if the cruise is rough or at the first sign of motion sickness. If the pills or the patch does not work and you are vomiting, then try a suppository such as Tigan, which should be in your first aid kit (page 27). If the vomiting persists longer than an hour after you have inserted the suppository, go to the medical facility. The health care providers will be able to give you an injection of Tigan or another medication to stop the vomiting. Depending on how long you have been vomiting, you might also need fluid replacement through an intravenous line. This can be done at the medical facility.

When you go to see the sights

Many cruise ships stop at different ports for passengers to go sightseeing. Pack a bag of necessities when you go. Be sure to take your blood glucose meter, insulin or diabetes pills, and any other medications you will need while you are gone. Take a snack (such as cheese and crackers or half a sandwich) with you and glucose to treat low blood sugar. And pack at least one bottle of water. Put on suntan lotion before you leave and take some with you. Take your sunglasses and a sun hat. Be sure to wear good walking shoes. Carry your letter that says you have diabetes and need to carry your blood glucose meter, lancets, and, if needed, syringes. You should always wear a medic alert ID.

The cruise director should be able to tell you about places to eat safely while you are sightseeing. Leave enough time to get back to the ship, so you are not left at port!

CRUISE SHIP CHECKLIST

(Keep these things with you on board ship and
at ports of call)

☐ Blood glucose monitoring supplies

☐ Insulin for the day

☐ Insulin cool pack

☐ Other medications as needed

☐ Glucose tablet or other quick-acting glucose

☐ Suntan lotion

☐ Sunglasses

☐ Sun hat

☐ Comfortable shoes and socks

☐ Medic alert ID on person and supplies

☐ Dramamine (pills) or Scopolamine (patches) for
motion sickness

☐ Snacks

☐ Bottle of water

☐ Letter indicating that you have diabetes and need
to carry blood glucose supplies, insulin and other
supplies with you (Appendix 1-B)

Eating Well and Exercise on the Road

6

Eating well while traveling and being away from home can be challenging. You'll need to give some thought to time changes, availability of food, variety of food, how food is prepared, and portion sizes. Unless you have a kitchen and you can prepare some of your meals, you will be eating out for all three meals, so it's time to sharpen your eating-out skills. This chapter has suggestions to help you choose wisely from a variety of cuisines. To balance the blood glucose effect of the delicious (we hope) meals that you will be having, travel also offers an abundance of opportunities to get much more exercise than you usually do.

Time changes

It is best to get yourself accustomed to the time zone you are visiting as quickly as possible. If you go to bed, get up, and eat your meals based on the time where you are, you will adjust more quickly. But it may not be quite that simple. In some countries, it is customary to eat meals at a later time. Or the big

103

meal of the day is the noon meal rather than the evening meal. You can make adjustments for this. If you take insulin or oral medication specifically for the dinner meal, but you will be eating your larger meal at the noon hour, consider taking your rapid-acting or short-acting insulin before the noon meal instead. If you are on an insulin pump, simply switch the dinner insulin program with the lunchtime insulin program. The same would be true of the oral medication designed to cover just your dinner meal. See Appendix 6-A for more about making adjustments to your medication for time changes, and discuss them with your health care practitioners.

If your dinner will be served several hours later than you usually eat, you may need to have your bedtime snack at the time you would ordinarily have dinner. Then you eat dinner later and probably will not need another snack. But don't guess; check your blood glucose before bed to see if you need a snack.

Where will you eat?

When you arrive at your destination, check out the availability of grocery stores, markets, and restaurants or other places to eat. Find out how far you will need to travel to get to these places and what transportation you can use to get there. Also ask about the hours of operation. For example, over the Easter weekend in European countries, all the grocery stores are closed for several days.

When you go out to eat, carry your blood glucose meter and insulin or diabetes pills with you. Do not take your insulin or other medications until you are sure when your food will be served. You might want to wait until the food is actually on the table before taking your medication

What will you eat?

Most restaurants offer a wide variety of foods. You can usually get the carbohydrates you need from breads, pasta, rice, potatoes, and fruit. Do not hesitate to ask questions about how dishes are prepared or about serving sizes. This is part of the service that you are paying for. Ask how foods are prepared. Ask about low-fat or fat-free salad dressings. (Be aware that fat-free salad dressings may have more carbohydrate than the regular dressing, so they will have an effect on your blood sugar, especially if you have several servings.)

You may request to have your foods prepared in a way different from what is listed on the menu. Fried foods can be broiled. Sauces and gravies can be served on the side. You will want to know if a sauce has sugar in it or is high in fat, because these ingredients will affect your blood sugar. Ask questions and you will help your waiter or waitress learn a little about diabetes, too.

Today, more and more people eat out at restaurants. Restaurant owners have become more health-conscious, and most menus have "lite" or "healthy" entrees. Most eating places offer sugar substitutes, diet beverages, fruit juice, and decaffeinated coffee and tea. Some have reduced-calorie salad dressings, low-fat or fat-free milk, and salt substitutes. But even if they don't offer special meals, it is pretty easy to find salads, fish and seafood, vegetables, baked or broiled food, and whole-grain breads. See Appendix 6-B for more suggestions for healthy food choices.

How much will you eat?

More often than not, restaurants serve really large portions. This is too much food for most people. You may be able to order a half portion or share your entree with a friend or family member. Look at your meal when it arrives. Before you begin to eat, decide how much of the food on your plate meets your real needs. Do not be afraid to leave food on your plate.

Nowadays, more restaurants are offering menus that list calories and nutrients or they can provide this information when you request it. If you ask, chefs can sometimes create low-fat entrees just for you. Some cooks will remove the skin from a chicken, omit extra butter on the dish, broil instead of fry, and serve sauces on the side. There are restaurants that will allow you to order small portions at reduced prices. All these improvements make it easier to fit restaurant foods into your meal plan.

Following the plan

You want to feel healthy and energized on your trip, so it's a good idea to try to follow your meal plan as much as possible. Here are some tips to help you.

- If you can, pick a restaurant that offers a wide variety of choices.

- If you don't know the ingredients in a dish or the serving size, ask.

- Try to eat the same size servings that you eat at home.

- Ask that fish or meat be broiled with little added fat.

- Ask to have sour cream or butter for the baked potato on the side or not brought at all.

- If you are on a low-sodium diet or want to cut back, ask that no or little salt be added to your food.

- Ask to have sauces, gravy, and dressings served on the side.

- Avoid breaded or fried foods. If the food arrives breaded, you can peel off the outer coating or send it back if you ordered it without breading.

- Use the menu creatively. For instance, order the fruit cup appetizer or the breakfast melon for your dessert after dinner.

- Ask for substitutions, such as low-fat cottage cheese, baked potato instead of French fries, or a double portion of a vegetable instead of the fries.

- Ask about low-calorie items, such as salad dressings, even if they are not listed on the menu. Remember, you are the customer; it is okay to ask for what you need.

What about fast foods?

Today fast food restaurants are offering healthier choices, such as salads, baked potatoes, chili, and grilled chicken, that make it easier to fit fast food into a healthy eating plan. But there are still plenty of high-fat, high-calorie fast food choices, so take care with what you order. It is possible to eat an entire day's worth of fat, salt, and calories in just one fast food meal.

Follow the guidelines your dietitian or health care provider has given you. For instance, you may be counting calories or grams of carbohydrate or grams of fat. If you have not been given guidelines, try to keep these points in mind:

1. eat a variety of foods in medium-sized amounts

2. eat more vegetables

3. limit your fat intake

4. watch the amount of sodium in the food choices

Many fast food restaurants can give you the nutritional information on their foods if you ask. By knowing the nutritional value of the fast food, you can choose ones that will fit into your meal plan. If you have some higher-fat fast food for one meal, try to eat low-fat foods like fruits and vegetables for your other meals that day. Balance is important. Here are some tips to help you choose among fast foods.

- For breakfast, try a plain bagel, toast, or English muffin. Drink fruit juice or low-fat milk. Order cold cereal with skim milk, pancakes without butter, or plain scrambled eggs. Limit or pass up the bacon and sausage.

- Load up on lettuce and vegetables at a salad bar. Go easy on the dressing, bacon bits, cheeses, croutons, mayonnaise, and macaroni salads. Too much of even a low-calorie salad dressing can make a difference. Check the number of calories on the packet.

- Order regular (or junior-size) sandwiches rather than the jumbo, giant, or deluxe sandwiches to get fewer calories and less fat, cholesterol, and sodium.

- Choose lean roast beef, turkey or chicken breast, or lean ham sandwiches.

- Skip the buttery croissant and eat your sandwich on a bun or bread instead to save calories and fat.

- Choose chicken or fish if it is roasted, unbreaded, grilled, baked, or broiled without fat. Chicken or fish that is battered, breaded, or fried is higher in calories and fat than a hamburger.

- Stay away from double burgers or super hot dogs with cheese, chili, or sauces. Cheese can carry an extra 100 calories, as well as extra fat and sodium.

- Order items without toppings, rich sauces, or mayonnaise. Add lettuce, tomato, onion, and mustard instead.

- Choose cheese pizza with vegetables. Toppings such as pepperoni, sausage, and extra cheese add calories, fat, and sodium. A word of caution: the high carbohydrate content of pizza can make blood glucose levels go really high in some people, but the high fat content of pizza may delay the blood glucose rise until several hours later. Check your blood glucose at different times after eating pizza to learn how it affects you.

- Order tacos, tostados, bean burritos, soft tacos, and other non-fried items in Mexican restaurants.

Choose chicken over beef. Avoid beans refried in lard. Pile on extra lettuce, tomatoes, and salsa. Go easy on cheese, sour cream, and guacamole. Watch out for the deep-fried taco salad shell; a taco salad can have more than 1,000 calories!

■ If you have room for dessert, go for sugar-free nonfat frozen yogurt. Ices, sorbets, and sherbets do have less fat and fewer calories than ice cream. But they are full of sugar and can send your blood glucose too high unless you work the extra sugar into your meal plan. Some fast food places now offer fresh fruit!

By making the right choices and balancing the meals when you eat out, you can enjoy yourself and take care of your diabetes at the same time.

Physical activity

If you've done quite a bit of walking or physical activity during the day, be aware that it will continue to lower your blood glucose for hours. This is one of the glorious benefits of exercise. When you walk all day or do a lot of physical activity, you will need an extra snack between meals containing protein and carbohydrate, such as cheese and crackers or half a meat sandwich. If you are very active, you may want to decrease your diabetes medication to prevent low blood glucose. Use your glucose monitor to help you decide. And discuss this possibility with your health care provider before you go.

Exercise and insulin. If you are on insulin, eat a protein-and-carbohydrate snack as needed during the day, and first try lowering your insulin doses by 10%.

Check your blood glucose levels the first day of activity, and decide whether you need to lower your insulin the next day by an additional 10%. Be aware that the blood glucose–lowering effects of exercise may carry over into the night or the next day. Since you can't be sure how much your blood glucose levels will drop from increasing your activity level, go ahead and check your blood glucose more often. Always carry quick-acting carbohydrates, such as fruit juice or glucose tablets, with you to treat low blood sugar if it occurs. You may need a bedtime snack. It's healthier to lower your insulin dose than to have to worry about unexpected low blood sugar and then, have to eat to raise your blood glucose level.

Exercise and diabetes pills. If you are taking diabetes pills that can cause low blood glucose, you need to be aware of the effect that increased physical activity has on your blood glucose level, too. If you check your blood glucose and find it is low, eat a snack containing protein and carbohydrate. If you'll be hiking all day for example, you may need to eat several snacks over the day.

You might wonder whether you can lower your dose of medication. However, except for repaglinide (Prandin), acarbose (Precose), or miglitol (Glyset), making adjustments to your oral meds does not have an immediate effect on your blood sugar level. It is also more difficult to adjust oral meds than it is to lower insulin by a few units. Some diabetes pills may be cut in half. Check with your pharmacist about the pills you take. The problem is that cutting pills in half does not mean that you will get a correct dose, and it may alter the way your body is able to absorb and use the medication.

Most oral diabetes medications do come in a variety of dosages. Ask your health care provider about the smaller dose pills, and whether you might take them on the days you are very active. For instance, your dose of medication is a 10 mg pill at breakfast and 10 mg pill at dinner. That same medication may come in a 2.5 mg pill or a 5 mg pill. Request a prescription for the 2.5 mg pill. Instead of taking one 10 mg pill before breakfast and one 10 mg pill before dinner, you would take four 2.5 mg pills before breakfast and four 2.5 mg pills before dinner. Then on the days you are active and your blood glucose levels are running low, you could adjust your dosage by taking only three 2.5 mg pills before breakfast and three before dinner. You'll need to check your blood glucose frequently to help you decide whether you need to adjust your medication and how much.

Enjoy

The three Es of travel could well be eating, exercise, and enjoyment. With a little planning ahead, you can easily have all three. And create many pleasant memories of your trip.

Adjusting Diabetes Medications for Mealtime Changes

Present Program (Largest meal dinner)	Changes (Largest meal lunch)

INSULIN

Two injections daily

20 units NPH or lente at breakfast 10 units regular or Humalog at breakfast	No change
20 units NPH or lente at dinner 10 units regular or Humalog at dinner	10 units regular or Humalog at lunch 20 units NPH or lente at dinner

Three injections daily

20 units NPH or lente at breakfast 10 units regular or Humalog at breakfast	No change
10 units regular or Humalog at dinner	10 units regular or Humalog at lunch
20 units NPH or lente at bedtime	No change

Present Program (Largest meal dinner)	Changes (Largest meal lunch)
Four injections daily 20 units NPH or lente at breakfast 10 units regular or Humalog at breakfast	No change
10 units regular or Humalog at lunch	Take at dinner
14 units regular or Humalog at dinner	Take at lunch
20 units NPH or lente at bedtime	No change

INSULIN PUMP THERAPY

Switch bolus taken at dinner with bolus taken at lunch.

ORAL DIABETES MEDICATION

Continue to take as prescribed.

Healthy Choices for Eating Out

Green Light	Red Light
Appetizers	
Tomato juice, unsweetened juice	Sweetened juices
Clear broth, bouillon, consommé	Cream soups, thick soups
Raw vegetables	Marinated vegetables
Fresh fruit, unsweetened	Canned fruit cocktail
Fresh steamed seafood	Breaded or fried seafood
Eggs	
Poached or boiled	Fried, creamed, or scrambled
Salads	
Tossed vegetable	Coleslaw
Cottage cheese	Canned fruit or gelatin salads
Breads	
Whole-grain rolls, crackers Biscuits, breads	Sweet rolls, coffee cake, croissants
Potatoes, pasta, and rice	
Baked, boiled, or steamed potatoes	Fried, French fried, creamed, scalloped, or au gratin potatoes

Green Light	Red Light

Fats

| Low-calorie salad dressing | Regular salad dressing |
| Low-fat sour cream or yogurt | Regular sour cream
Gravy, cream sauces |

Vegetables

| Raw, stewed, steamed, or boiled | Creamed, scalloped, or au gratin |

Meat, poultry, and fish

| Roasted, baked, or broiled lean meats with skin or fat removed | Fried, battered, or breaded; cured meats; organ meats; stews and casseroles; gravy |

Desserts

| Fresh fruit or fruit juice
Nonfat or low-fat frozen yogurt | Sweetened fruit, pudding, custard, pastries |

Beverages

| Water, coffee, tea (decaffeinated)
Fat-free milk, diet soda, water | Chocolate milk, cocoa, milkshakes, regular soft drinks |

Illness During Your Trip 7

Taking precautions to prevent illness is the best way to stay healthy and enjoy your trip. However, if you do get sick, you need to be able to respond quickly and know when and where to seek help. You can pack medications to treat common illnesses, such as colds or diarrhea (pages 25–27). If you haven't already, talk with your provider about making a plan for sick-day care (see Appendix 7-A), and be sure to take it with you. When you arrive at your destination, find out where the nearest health care center and pharmacy are located. Contact the ADA at 1-800-DIABETES (1-800-342-2383) if you need help locating health care in the United States.

If you are traveling in a foreign country, call the U.S. Consulate or U.S. Embassy when you arrive (see Appendix 8-A). If you will be in the area for an extended period of time, give them your phone number and tell them how you can be reached. The primary job of the consular officer is to help U.S. citizens traveling abroad, so they can help you in many ways, especially if you become ill and need assistance. They have lists of doctors and health care facilities in the area.

What can you do before you go?

Before you travel to foreign countries, it's a good idea to schedule a travel medical interview at a travel health clinic. The interview and visit will address your travel-related needs. Based on where you will be traveling, the health care providers will advise you of health risks, the types of medications you should take with you, and any immunizations you need before you travel. Have this check-up several months before your trip. This will allow enough time for the travel clinic to review your medical history, order any needed tests, and give you any immunizations that you might need.

Immunizations. Most immunizations are given in a series over several months. Be sure to allow enough time to get the whole series. Before the visit, check your records to determine which immunizations you have had and when you got them. Also, know the date of your last tetanus shot. They are good for 10 years in adults, and this is a good time to update your tetanus if you need to.

Keep a record of all of your immunizations. The health clinic or your doctor can provide you a small booklet for recording the types of immunizations you have had and the dates you got them. When you travel, take a copy of your record with you. Keep the record of your immunizations with your important travel papers.

Be sure to have a flu shot each year. People with diabetes are four times more likely to die of complications of the flu or pneumonia than people who do not have diabetes. The vaccine may not prevent you from getting the flu, but it will minimize your symptoms and the length of your illness if you do get it. You should also get a pneumonia vaccine. After the initial vaccine, you should have a booster shot every 5–6 years.

Do you need to check your blood sugar when you are sick?

Yes. In fact, if you are ill, you need to check your blood glucose more frequently than usual. If you take insulin, you may need to increase your insulin to keep your blood glucose in the normal range. If your blood glucose is low because you are unable to eat, you may need to lower your insulin dose. Do not stop taking your insulin when you are ill. It is best to work out a sick-day plan with your provider or educator before you travel that will include how to make adjustments to your insulin (see Appendix 7-B).

What do you do when vomiting is part of the illness?

If you are ill and vomiting, you must be sure that you do not get dehydrated. You will need to take in fluids to prevent this from happening. You have to strike a careful balance because drinking fluids may cause more vomiting, but you must not let yourself get dehydrated. If you are vomiting, you will need to adjust your meal plan. Although you need carbohydrates to prevent low blood sugar, solid food will just aggravate the problem. You need fluids that contain carbohydrate.

You can try converting your meal plan into liquids. Check your blood glucose every 2 hours. If your blood glucose is greater than 240 mg/dl, sip fluids that are sugar free, and check for ketones. If your blood glucose is less than 240 mg/dl, then drink fluids with 15 g of carbohydrate in them (Appendix 7-C).

You may control vomiting with a rectal suppository, such as Tigan. This is a prescription item and should be part of your first aid kit (see pages 25–27). After you insert the Tigan, it usually begins to work in 30 minutes. Do not resume your normal meal plan yet. Continue to monitor your blood glucose every 2 hours and sip fluids. Most flu bugs will last 24–48 hours. Be sure the flu is over before you begin eating solid food again.

If, despite all of your efforts, you are unable to control the vomiting, you may become dehydrated. Then it may be necessary for you to go to a medical clinic or hospital to get fluids intravenously. If you are vomiting without relief for 6 hours, seek medical care.

What do you do if you have vomiting and diarrhea?

If you have the flu and are vomiting and also have diarrhea, you will not be able to use a rectal suppository such as Tigan. It will be important to check your blood glucose every 2 hours and to check for ketones (see pages 82–83). This is a serious situation. You must replace fluids to prevent becoming dehydrated.

If diarrhea is severe, taking medication such as Imodium can be helpful if you are able to take the medication without vomiting it up. If you have vomiting and diarrhea for 6 hours and you are unable to keep any fluids down, you should seek medical assistance right away.

Why do you need to check for ketones?

When you are ill, you must check your urine for ketones (pages 82–83). Ketones are an acid that is a by-product when the body burns fat for fuel instead of carbohydrate. If you take insulin, it means that you need more. If you take the diabetes pill metformin, it means that it is building up in your body and causing lactic acidosis. No matter which diabetes medication you take, if your body is producing ketones and you don't do anything about it, you can develop a very serious condition called diabetic ketoacidosis (DKA). It can lead to a life-threatening situation and usually requires a trip to the hospital.

Early signs of DKA include high blood glucose levels (higher than 240 mg/dl), moderate to large amounts of ketones in the urine or the blood, headache, muscle and joint aches, and stomach upset. You may only have high blood glucose and ketones, with no other symptoms. It is very important to treat the high blood glucose levels and ketones with insulin and lots of fluids. Usually with extra insulin, the blood glucose and ketone levels will come down. Check the ketone level hourly. If you are unable to lower the blood glucose and clear the ketones with insulin and fluids within 4 hours, seek medical attention. If you slip further into DKA, you may experience shortness of breath, chest pain, and vomiting. If you have these symptoms, you must seek medical care immediately.

What can you do about traveler's diarrhea?

One of your concerns when traveling outside of the United States is getting traveler's diarrhea—a great risk to your health. It usually comes from contact with bacteria-contaminated food or water. The best treatment is prevention. Always drink bottled water. Even brush your teeth with bottled water. Never use ice in drinks. Be sure food is completely cooked. If raw fruits and vegetables cannot be peeled, do not eat them. Do not eat raw vegetables.

If you will be traveling outside of the country, you may want to take Pepto Bismal daily or antibiotics to prevent traveler's diarrhea from occurring. The correct choice for you will depend on your health needs and where you will be traveling. Talk with your health care provider about this. These same medications are also the ones you would use to treat traveler's diarrhea if you got it (see Appendix 7-D).

Traveler's diarrhea can be categorized into three types. The first type, watery diarrhea, is characterized by explosive, non-bloody stools with nausea, vomiting, abdominal cramping, and fever. This type of diarrhea can affect as many as 60% of travelers. The second type is dysentery. Dysentery affects 15% of travelers. It is characterized by bloody, mucus-laden diarrhea, bowel inflammation, fever, and abdominal pain. Dysentery requires antibiotics and medical care.

The third type of traveler's diarrhea is chronic diarrhea. This accounts for fewer than 2% of all cases. Chronic diarrhea often lasts for several weeks. Symptoms include abdominal pain, bloating, fatigue, weight loss, and fever. You need medical evaluation and treatment for chronic diarrhea.

What can you do to avoid constipation?

Drink lots of water—not caffeine drinks such as tea or coffee because they are diuretics and remove water from your body. And not carbonated drinks because they deplete your body of water, too. Eat vegetables. Eat well-washed fruit with the skins on. Eat whole-grains such as brown rice. Eat some more vegetables. Avoid highly-refined foods with lots of white flour, sugar, and salt. Get some exercise. Take your bran flakes with you.

Should you be watching for any illness connected with wearing an insulin pump?

If you wear an insulin pump, there is a risk of irritation or infection at the insertion site of your infusion line. You can prevent most site infections by

- washing your hands
- using the sterile technique you have learned
- changing your infusion site every other day

If the site appears irritated when you remove the infusion line, apply warm compresses to the area. This increases circulation, which speeds healing. Be sure to insert your new infusion line in an area away from the irritated site. Check it regularly. It may take several days, but gradually, any redness or irritation should go away.

An infusion site may also become infected. An infected site is usually red, warm to the touch, or painful, and it may have drainage. Often the infected area will be hard to the touch. In addition to the care you would provide to an irritated site (keep it clean and apply warm compresses), you need an antibiotic.

You should pack an antibiotic that will treat site infections (see page 26). An infection will often cause high blood glucose levels. Check your blood sugar more frequently to see whether you will need to adjust your insulin. You may also need to check for ketones.

What do you pack for coughs and colds?

Be sure to pack medications for treating colds and coughs. Most over-the-counter cold medications are safe for people with diabetes to use. It is best to review this with your health care provider before you travel to be sure these medications will not interfere with other medications that you are taking. Sugar-free cough syrups are available over the counter and by prescription, but they may be difficult to find on the road. Put a bottle of cough syrup in your first aid kit.

What can you do about jet lag?

Jet lag can occur if you are crossing multiple time zones. It occurs when you are flying east or west, not north or south. The quick change in time zones does not allow your body to adjust to the new time schedule. You may experience headaches, constipation, insomnia, nervousness, irritability, sluggishness, and forgetfulness.

There are a few things that you can do to minimize jet lag. Try to arrive at your destination at bedtime. Get yourself on the schedule of your destination as quickly as possible. Get plenty of rest the day before your departure and when you arrive. Sleep during your flight. Avoid alcohol and caffeine. Drink fluids to avoid becoming dehydrated because this can make the symptoms of jet lag worse. Drink one 8-oz non-alcoholic, decaffeinated beverage every hour of your flight.

What is a UTI and what can you do about it?

People with diabetes are more prone to urinary track infections (UTIs). Keeping your blood glucose levels well controlled can help prevent UTIs because this allows the body's immune system to ward off bacteria that may enter the urinary track system. However, UTIs may be caused by another condition. Over time, the muscles of the bladder may become affected by nerve changes caused by diabetes in a condition called neurogenic bladder.

The nerve damage to the bladder does not allow the bladder to empty completely when you urinate. The urine left in the bladder may become contaminated by bacteria. If you have more than two UTIs a year, you will need to see a urologist, a doctor specializing in disease of the urinary track. Neurogenic bladder can be treated with medications, so the bladder can empty properly and infections can be prevented.

The symptoms of a UTI are:

- cloudy or bloody urine

- pain when you urinate

- a constant feeling of pressure and needing to urinate

These symptoms need to be treated with antibiotics. If possible, get a urine culture at a health care clinic before you start taking an antibiotic. The urinalysis will help the health care provider determine the best antibiotic for the bacteria in your urine.

If you are unable to get a culture, start taking the antibiotic in your first aid kit. It should be a broad-spectrum antibiotic that kills the usual bacteria that grow in the bladder. For the first 24–48 hours of treatment of a UTI, you often feel pain when you try to urinate. The pain is caused by a contraction or spasm of the urethra, the tube through which urine comes out of the body. If you have this pain, you will want to take, in addition to the antibiotic, a prescription medication called Pyridum. Keep a supply of these tablets in your first aid kit (pages 25–27). Pyridum will stop the spasms of the urethra and work as a local anesthetic on the pain. Pyridum will turn the urine a dark red-orange color. In women, it may stain underwear, but a small sanitary pad can help if that is a problem. If you do not have any Pyridum, try urinating in a bathtub filled with clear warm water. This may also decrease the discomfort until the antibiotics have started to work.

Be sure to take all of the antibiotic even if you start feeling better. Starting today, drink at least eight glasses of water per day. Be sure to urinate whenever you have the urge. After you complete the antibiotics, get a urine culture done to be sure the bacteria is gone.

Some people find that drinking cranberry juice is helpful in preventing and treating bladder infections. If you drink a glass of cranberry juice, remember to count the amount of carbohydrate in the juice when you are figuring out how much of your diabetes medication to take. If this works for you, there are also cranberry capsules you can take.

What can you do about vaginal infections?

Women with diabetes are more likely to get vaginal infections. Vaginal infections can cause pain, itching, and a discharge from the vaginal area. Controlling your blood glucose will help minimize these infections. There are several over-the-counter medications to treat vaginal infections, such as Monistat cream or suppositories, that you can take with you on your trip. If the symptoms do not cease or they come back, be sure to seek medical assistance.

Can you arrange for health care before you go?

Check with your health insurance company to see what coverage they will give you on your trip. Be sure you find out the restrictions and requirements, and everything that is covered including paying for flying you home. Medicare does not cover you for overseas travel. If your health insurance does not cover you on your trip, there are many emergency services to help you with health care while traveling (Appendix 7-E). Some require you to become a member before you can obtain their services, but most just charge a fee if you need care. Be sure to contact the agencies before beginning your trip, so you are familiar with the services each of them offers.

You can buy special trip insurance that also covers health care during the trip and a change in flight or cruise schedule to return home. Most have toll-free hotlines, assist you with finding a physician, pay for medical care, and arrange for getting you home. Some of the companies that offer travel and health insurance are Access America (1-800-284-8300), International SOS Assistance (1-800-523-8930), Assist-Card (1-800-874-2223), and Travelex Insurance Services (1-800-228-9792). You must tell the company that you have diabetes and get in writing what they will cover for you and what they will not. For example, Assist-Card can provide translation services and send a doctor to your hotel room if you are sick, cover medical or dental care, and offers accidental death insurance among other services.

You may already have a credit card that covers illness and special or medical care while you are traveling when you charge the trip on the card. For example, the Platinum American Express card or a Gold MasterCard often covers these costs and the costs of having you airlifted home. Call your credit card company to see what travel benefits you may have.

Sick-Day Care

What to do if you are too sick to eat:

1. Measure your blood glucose every 2 hours and record the result.

2. Call your health care provider for assistance. If you are unable to reach him or her, take at least half your dose of insulin.

3. Drink fluids every 2 hours. Select fluids from the choices listed below and sip them slowly over a 2-hour period. Use ice chips; you may tolerate this fluid better.

   - 1 cup (8 oz) regular soda (not diet soda)

   - 1 cup (8 oz) fruit juice

   - 2 cups (16 oz) Gatorade

   - Sweetened tea (2 level tsp sugar in 1 cup tea)

AND

   - In addition to the above items, 1 cup of bouillon or (dried) chicken soup, with water

4. Drink additional water during the day or use ice chips to avoid dehydration.

5. Seek health care when:

   - Your blood glucose is 240 mg/dl or more and does not drop below 200 mg/dl when you use additional insulin

- Your blood glucose is 240 mg/dl or more and there are ketones in your urine

- You feel too sick to eat, are unable to keep down food or fluids, and you feel you need help or advice

If you take diabetes pills, do not stop taking them. Ask your provider whether you should adjust the dosage for sick days.

- Check your blood glucose levels more often—every 2 hours.

- Check for ketones if your blood glucose is 240 mg/dl or more.

- Use the food choices on page 130.

Insulin Supplements for Sick Days

When you are sick, you may need more insulin. Your blood sugar levels will begin to rise. To compensate for this problem you will need to add extra regular or lispro (Humalog) insulin to your usual doses of insulin until your blood glucose levels return to normal. The dose of extra insulin is based on your blood glucose levels, so you must use your blood glucose meter. If you have ketones in your urine or blood, you'll need to double the dose of insulin listed below. Take the extra insulin before each meal, or if you are not eating meals, take it every 4 hours. Do not take extra insulin before bed because it could cause low blood glucose problems while you are asleep.

Be sure to measure your blood glucose every 2 hours. If your blood glucose is higher than 240 mg/dl, check your urine or blood for ketones. Keep a record of your blood glucose levels, ketone levels, your usual dose of insulin, and any extra insulin you take. Record the time, too.

For blood glucose of	Add to normal insulin dose
Less than 200	0 units of regular or Humalog
200–249	2 units of regular or Humalog
250–299	3 units of regular or Humalog
300–349	4 units of regular or Humalog
350–399	5 units of regular or Humalog
400 or more	6 units of regular or Humalog

Double the extra dose of insulin if you have ketones present.

Adapted from "Sick Days," page 75, *Diabetes 101*, Brackenridge et al.

Fluids to Drink when You Are Ill

Be sure to contact your health care facility if you are having trouble eating or keeping foods down, and keep taking your insulin. The following is a list of foods that are easy to digest and may be helpful when you are feeling ill. Since you have taken your insulin, you should take some carbohydrate every 2 hours throughout the day and night. The foods listed below each contain 15 g of carbohydrate.

Apple juice	1/2 cup
Grape juice	1/3 cup
Orange juice	1/2 cup
Gatorade	1 1/2 cup
Applesauce	1/2 cup
Cooked cereal	1/2 cup
Baked custard	1/2 cup
Saltines	6
Fruited yogurt	1/2 cup
Ice cream	1/2 cup
Pineapple juice	1/2 cup
Popsicle	1/2
Jello	1/3 cup
Thick soup	1/2 cup
Thin soup	1 cup
Regular soda	1/2 cup
Honey	3 tsp
Lifesavers	7
Milk	1 cup

MENU

8 AM _____

10 AM _____

12 noon _____

2 PM _____

4 PM _____

6 PM _____

8 PM _____

10 PM _____

You'll need extra fluids (calorie free) to prevent dehydration. Use free liquids such as broth or water.

Medications to Prevent and Treat Traveler's Diarrhea

Dose	Dosage	
	For Prevention	For Treatment
*Bismuth subsalicylate (Pepto Bismal)	2 tablets or 30 ml 4 times per day	2 tablets or 30 ml every hour (don't exceed 8 doses/24 hrs)
**Ciprofloxacin (Cipro)	500 mg per day	500 mg twice daily for 3 days
**Ofloxacin	400 mg per day	400 mg twice daily for 3 days
**Loperamide	Not indicated	4 mg to start, then 2 mg after each unformed stool (not to exceed 16 mg/24 hrs)

There are also other medications to treat traveler's diarrhea. Discuss with your health care provider which ones are best for you to use.
* Over-the-counter medication; no prescription needed.
** Prescription medication.

APPENDIX 7-E

Emergency Assistance

Overseas Citizens' Emergency Center
2201 C Street NW
Washington, DC 20520
1-202-647-5225

International Association for Medical Assistance to Travelers

417 Center Street
Lewiston, NY 14092
1-716-754-4883

Free service. Members receive a directory of English-speaking physicians in 125 countries who will provide 24-hour care at reasonable fees.

American Express Global Assistance Service
United States: 1-800-554-2639
Abroad (call collect): 1-202-783-7474

Provides emergency assistance to card members if more than 100 miles from home. The hotline will refer you to a nearby legal or medical professional, will arrange for a translator, and notify your home or office.

Assist-Card
1001 South Bayshore Drive, Suite 2302
Miami, FL 33131
1-800-874-2223

International assistance ranging from medical and dental to concierge services. Provides assistance within the U.S. for foreign visitors.

Hoteldocs
1-800-468-3537

Sends an American Medical Association–recruited doctor to your U.S. hotel room within 40 minutes of your call, at any time of day.

International SOS Assistance, Inc.
P.O. Box 11568
Philadelphia, PA 19116
1-215-244-1500
1-800-523-8930

Provides emergency assistance to members. If medical assistance cannot be rendered locally, the traveler will be evacuated to a place with medical facilities.

Travel Guard International
1145 Clark Street
Stevens Point, WI 54481
1-715-345-0505

Talk to your travel agent about this service. Offers a 24-hour emergency claims service, emergency assistance, medical expenses, baggage and travel documents coverage, and trip-cancellation insurance. Underwritten by the Insurance Company of North America.

Travelex Insurance Services
11717 Burt Street, Ste. 202
Omaha, NE 68154-1500
1-800-228-9792

Planning for Special Situations

You can travel wherever you want to go. The key is to plan ahead, so you can be prepared. Try to anticipate problems that may occur and always do the following:

- Know who to call in an emergency.

- Pack enough supplies to be able to manage your diabetes.

- Pack enough food for 24 hours or more, depending on where you're going.

Overseas travel

Foreign travel can be a challenge if you have not planned ahead. There are United States Consulates in more than 140 countries around the world. They are there to help you, so use them as a resource. Before you travel, contact them either by telephone or through their website (Appendix 8-A) for information regarding your travel destination. The information sheets include country description, entry requirements, customs regulations, crime information, medical facilities, medical insurance, immunization requirements, and how to register at the U.S. Consulate when you arrive.

Foreign languages

If you do not speak the language of the country you are visiting, try to learn a few key phrases before you go. You may need to know how to say: I have diabetes, I need sugar, I need a doctor. Appendix 8-B at the end of this chapter has helpful sentences in Spanish, German, French, Italian, Russian, Japanese, and Chinese. If you photocopy the sentences or write them down and take them with you, you can read them or point to them if you don't feel you can say them. You may want to also take a dictionary or language book with you for help translating other phrases. Ask the concierge or desk clerk at your hotel to write out the address and phone number of the hotel. You can show the address to a taxi driver, or if you are lost, it will assist you in getting back to your hotel.

Always take these along

There are several things to always carry with you:

- your insulin or diabetes pills
- blood glucose monitor and supplies
- foods to treat low blood glucose
- at least one snack (preferably two or three)

If you need to treat low blood glucose, you do not want to be wandering around looking for a place that has something safe for you to eat. In your cooler or tote bag, also keep the letter that explains why you are carrying these supplies (see Appendix 1-B).

Camping

Camping can be a fun way to vacation. Whether you are camping in warm or cold weather, you will need to take special precautions with your insulin. Placing insulin in a cooler will work, but be sure it does not touch the ice. The insulin can freeze and lose potency. If you are camping outdoors in cold weather, don't leave your insulin outside. You can place it in a cooler or a wide-mouth insulated thermos. The thermos will keep it at a steady temperature. Or you can tuck the insulin into your sleeping bag with you, so it won't freeze.

If you are cold, your blood sugar may fall. Pay attention to your symptoms and don't guess; go ahead and check your blood sugar level. If you are hiking at higher altitudes, be aware that the symptoms of high altitude sickness (which for people accustomed to living at sea level can occur as low as 9,000 feet) are sometimes similar to the symptoms of low blood sugar. You also need to know that being at a higher altitude can affect the way your blood glucose meter works. If you know you're going to high altitudes, call your meter company before you go and ask how to adjust your meter to get the correct results under the new conditions.

Keep all of your diabetes supplies and a complete first aid kit (pages 25–27) in waterproof containers. This will keep them dry, clean, and out of the way of animals and insects. Bring plenty of clothes suitable for the climate—highs and lows. Remember that wherever you go, even in the desert, nights often get cool.

Bring extra shoes and socks to change into if yours get wet. If you will be swimming, wear water shoes to protect your feet from injury and infection. In fact, never go barefoot, even in your tent.

Pack a cellular phone for emergencies. Know the phone number and where the nearest emergency center is located.

Use insect repellent to protect yourself from insect bites. Try it out at home to be sure you will not have an allergic reaction or skin irritation to the repellent.

Use sunscreen, a sun hat, sunglasses, and lightweight long-sleeved clothing to protect you from the sun. After-sun creams with aloe or vitamin E are helpful if you have had too much sun.

If you will be hiking, biking, swimming, or getting more exercise than usual, you should check your blood glucose more often because exercise lowers your blood glucose for hours afterward, even into the next day. So after quite a bit of exercise, measure your blood glucose before each meal and at bedtime. Always carry something with you to treat low blood glucose (see Appendix 3-A). You may need to take less insulin or adjust the dosage of your diabetes pill or eat some carbohydrate-containing food to balance the beneficial effect exercise has on your blood sugar (see pages 81–82). Be sure your companions know your symptoms of low blood sugar and what to do if you experience a low, including how to use the glucagon kit.

Long trips to the wilderness

Long trips to remote areas require serious planning, but they can be —and have been—done by people with diabetes! In addition to the health visits, immunizations, and supplies, you must know the area you will be traveling in. Talk with others who have done the same or similar trips. Talk with the company or travel agency that will be setting up the trip. Learn from others what to expect when you get there. Some of the questions you need to ask are:

- What facilities will be available?

- Where will you be staying?

- How will you obtain food?

- What types of food are available?

- Will there be storage available for your insulin?

- What medical facilities are available?

- What assistance can you expect if a medical emergency occurs?

Many of these trips are so remote that you may not see anyone except the people you are traveling with for long periods of time. All of these questions need to be answered before you take such a trip. And at least one of your companions needs to know how to recognize and treat low blood sugar, including how to use a glucagon kit.

After your questions are answered, it is time to plan what you will need to take with you. All the advice for general traveling tips apply. The difference is that you have no way to obtain more diabetes supplies if something happens to yours. Take great care in packing and handling your diabetes supplies (in several bags) and keep them with you. It will be important to pack snacks that you can divide into single servings and seal so that they do not attract animals or insects.

Scuba diving

Scuba diving is a favorite pastime of many people who visit warm tropical areas. There is no reason that you cannot learn to scuba dive. First, you need to take a course and become certified in scuba diving. Then, there are several precautions that you need to follow to make diving safe.

- Always dive with a partner who knows you have diabetes and knows how to treat low blood glucose.

- Check blood glucose 2–3 times before each dive.

Your blood glucose should be above 150 mg/dl. If blood glucose is less than 150 mg/dl or dropping, take 5 g of glucose (Appendix 3-A) for every 25 mg/dl it is below 150 mg/dl. You and your dive partner should both carry liquid or gel glucose in a tube during every dive. Agree on a low blood sugar signal. Be very aware that swimming in cold water will cause your blood glucose to drop quickly, so be alert to symptoms of low blood glucose. Don't drink alcohol for 24 hours before the time of the dive.

Be sure to take your diving certification card when you travel. When you complete an application, you will be asked about your diabetes. Bring along a letter from your health care provider indicating their recommendations for you to be able to dive safely (Appendix B-C).

SCUBA DIVING GUIDELINES

1. The dive should follow a meal. Always measure your blood glucose several times before you dive. It should be at least 150 mg/dl and not dropping.

2. If your blood glucose before the dive is lower than 150 mg/dl, you need to eat or drink 5 g of glucose (5 g carbohydrate) for every 25 mg/dl it is below 150 mg/dl. Try carbohydrates such as milk, fruit juice, or glucose tablets or liquid.

3. You and your diving partner must carry liquid glucose or gel during the dive and use it as needed.

4. Measure your blood glucose right after the dive and eat or drink more carbohydrates if you need them.

5. Always dive with a companion who understands how to recognize and treat low blood sugar. Before you're under water, decide on a way to communicate that you may be developing low blood sugar.

6. You should have good blood glucose control during the days you plan to dive.

7. Don't drink alcohol in the 24 hours before diving or during diving activities.

APPENDIX 8-A

Consular Information Sheets

You can obtain a fax copy of Consular Information Sheets for foreign countries by dialing 1-202-647-3000 and entering the appropriate code or by visiting the State Department's Website at http://travel.state.gov.

Afghanistan	2344	Bosnia and	
Albania	2475	Herzegovina	2676
Algeria	2543	Botswana	2687
Andorra	2636	Brazil	2729
Angola	2646	British Virgin	
Antigua and		Islands	27481
Barbuda	2684	British West	
Argentina	2743	Indies	27482
Armenia	2763	Brunei	2786
Australia	28781	Bulgaria	2854
Azerbaijan	2937	Burkina Faso	2875
Bahamas	2242	Burundi	28783
Bahrain	2247	Cambodia	22621
Bangladesh	2264	Cameroon	2263
Barbados	2272	Canada	22622
Belarus	2352	Cape Verde	2273
Belgium	2354	Central Africa	
Belize	23542	Republic	2368
Benin	2364	Chad	2423
Bermuda	2376	Chile	2445
Bhutan	2488	China	2446
Bolivia	2654	Colombia	2656
		Comoros Islands	2666

Congo	2664	Ghana	4426
Costa Rica	2678	Gibraltar	4427
Cote d'Ivoire	2683	Greece	47331
Croatia	2762	Greenland	47332
Cuba	2822	Grenada	4736
Cyprus	2977	Guatemala	4828
Czech Republic	2932	Guinea	48461
Denmark	3366	Guinea-Bissau	48462
Djibouti	3542	Guyana	4892
Dominica	36641	Haiti	4248
Dominican Republic	36642	Honduras	4663
		Hong Kong	4664
East Jerusalem, West Bank and Gaza	3278	Hungary	4864
		Iceland	4235
		India	4634
Ecuador and Galapagos Islands	3282	Indonesia	4636
Egypt	3497	Iran	4726
El Salvador	3572	Iraq	4727
Equatorial Guinea	3782	Ireland	4735
Eritrea	3748	Israel	4772
Estonia	3786	Italy	4825
Ethiopia	3844	Jamaica	5262
Fiji	3454	Japan	5272
Finland	3465	Jordan	5673
France	3726	Kazakstan	5292
French Polynesia	37361	Kenya	5369
French West Indies	37362	Kuwait	5892
Gabon	4226	Kyrgyzstan	5974
Gambia	4262	Laos	5267
Georgia	4367	Latvia	5288
Germany	4376	Lebanon	5322

Lesotho	5376	Nicaragua	6422
Libya	5429	Niger	64431
Lithuania	5484	Nigeria	64432
Luxembourg	5893	North Korea	6678
Macau	6222	Norway	6679
Macedonia	6223	Oman	6626
Madagascar	6232	Pakistan	7254
Malawi	62521	Palau	7252
Malaysia	62522	Panama	7262
Maldives	6253	Papua New Guinea	7278
Mali	6254	Paraguay	7272
Malta	6258	Peru	7378
Marshall Islands	6277	Philippines	7445
Mauritania	62871	Poland	7652
Mauritius	62872	Portugal	7678
Mexico	6394	Qatar	7282
Micronesia	6427	Romania	76621
Moldova	6653	Russia	7877
Monaco	6662	Rwanda	7926
Mongolia	6664	Sao Tome and	
Morocco	6676	Principe	7268
Mozambique	6692	Saudi Arabia	7283
Myanmar	6926	Senegal	7363
Namibia	6264	Serbia and	
Nauru	62873	Montenegro	7372
Nepal	6372	Seychelles	7392
Netherlands	63841	Sierra Leone	7437
Netherlands		Singapore	7464
Antilles	63842	Slovak Republic	75681
New Zealand	6399	Slovenia	75682
		Solomon Islands	7656

Somalia	76622	Trinidad and Tobago	8746
South Africa	76881	Tunisia	8864
South Korea	76882	Turkey	88751
Spain	7724	Turkmenistan	88752
Sri Lanka	7745	Uganda	8426
St. Kitts and Nevis	7854	Ukraine	8572
St. Vincent and the Grenadines	7884	United Arab Emirates	86481
Sudan	7832	United Kingdom	86482
Surinam	7874	Uruguay	8784
Swaziland	7929	Uzbekistan	8923
Sweden	7933	Vanuatu	8268
Switzerland	7948	Venezuela	8363
Syria	7974	Vietnam	8438
Taiwan	8249	Western Samoa	9378
Tajikistan	8254	Yemen	9363
Tanzania (Zanzibar)	8269	Zaire	9247
Thailand	8424	Zambia	9262
Togo	8646	Zimbabwe	9462
Tonga	8664		

Foreign Language Phrases

Spanish

Please help me. I have diabetes.
Por favór ayudenme. Tengo diabetes.

May I please have some sugar or
fruit juice or Coke?
**¿Me podría asistir con azúcar, o
jugo de frutas, o una coca-cola?**

My blood sugar is too low.
Mi nivél de azúcar está muy bajo.

I must have something to eat.
Necesito comer algo con urgencia.

Where is the American Consulate?
¿Donde está el Consulado Americano?

Where is the hospital?
¿Donde está el hospital?

Where may I buy medicine?
¿Donde podría comprar medicina?

Where is the grocery store?
¿Donde está el mercado?

Where is a telephone?
¿Donde está el teléfono?

Where is the _____ Hotel?
¿Donde está el Hotel _____ ?

Where may I buy batteries?
¿Donde podría comprar baterias?

I need some milk to drink.
Necesito tomar leche.

I need to buy some insulin.
Necesito comprar insulina.

I need to buy some insulin syringes.
Necesito comprar jeringas.

German

Please help me. I have diabetes.
Helfen Sie mir bitte, ich bin ein Diabetiker.

May I please have some sugar or fruit juice or Coke?
Koennten Sie mir bitte etwas Zucker, einen Fruchtesaft oder eine Cola geben?

My blood sugar is too low.
Mein Blutzucker ist zu niedrig.

I must have something to eat.
Ich muss etwas zu essen haben.

Where is the American Consulate?
Wo ist das Amerikanische Konsulat?

Where is the hospital?
Wo ist das Hospital?

Where may I buy medicine?
Wo kann ich Medikamente einkaufen?

Where is the grocery store?
Wo ist ein Lebensmittelgeschaeft?

Where is the telephone?
Wo ist ein Telefon?

Where is the _____ Hotel?
Wo ist das _____ Hotel?

Where may I buy batteries?
Wo gibt es Batterien zu kaufen?

I need some milk to drink.
Koennten Sie mir bitte etwas milch geben?

I need to buy some insulin.
Ich muss das Insulin kaufen.

Can I buy diabetic supplies?
Kann ich diabetiker bedorf kaufen?

French

Please help me. I have diabetes.
Aidez-moi. Je suis diabetique.

May I please have some sugar or fruit juice or Coke?
Pouvez vous me donner du sucre, un jus de fruit ou un Coca Cola ?

My blood sugar is too low.
Mon taux de sucre dans le sang est trop bas. Je suis en etat d'hypoglycemie.

I must have something to eat.
Je dois manger quelque chose.

I need some milk to drink.
J'ai besoin de boire du lait.

I need to buy some insulin.
J'ai besoin d'acheter de l'insuline.

I need to buy some insulin syringes.
J'ai besoin d'acheter des seringues pour l'insuline.

Where is the American Consulate?
Ou se trouve le consulat des Etats-Unis?

Where is the hospital?
Ou se trouve l'hopital?

Where may I buy medicine?
Ou puis-je acheter des medicaments?
Ou est la pharmacie?

Where is the grocery store?
Ou est le supermarché?

Where is the telephone?
Ou est le téléphone?

Where is the _____ Hotel?
Ou est l'_____ hotel?

Where may I buy batteries?
Ou puis-je acheter des piles?

Italian

Please help me. I have diabetes.
Aiutatemi-ho il diabete. Soffro il diabete.

May I please have some sugar or
fruit juice or Coke?
**Per favore potrei avere un po' di
zucchero, un succo di frutta o
una coca cola?**

My blood sugar is too low.
Ho la glicemia troppo bassa.

I must have something to eat.
Devo mangiare qualcosa.

I need some milk to drink.
Devo bere del latte.

I need to buy some insulin.
Devo comprare la insulina per il diabete.

I need to buy some insulin syringes.
Mi occorrono le siringhe da insulina.

Where is the American Consulate?
Dov'è il consolato americano?

Where is the hospital?
Dov'è l'ospedale?

Where may I buy medicine?
Where is a pharmacy?
**Dov'è posso comprare della medicina?
Dov'è una farmacia?**

Where is the grocery store?
Dov'è un supermercato o un negozio alimentare?

Where is the telephone?
Dov'è c'è un telefono?

Where is the _____ Hotel?
Dov'è l'albergo _____ ?

Where may I buy batteries?
Dov'è posso comprare le pile?

Russian

Please help me. I have diabetes.
Помогите мне, пожалуйста.
Я диабетик.

May I please have some sugar or
fruit juice or Coke?
Можно сахар, сок или лимонад.

My blood sugar is too low.
У меня низкий уровень сахара в
крови.

I must have something to eat.
Мне надо поесть.

Where is the American Consulate?
Где американское консульство?

Where is the hospital?
Где больница?

Where may I buy medicine?
Где купить лекарство?

Where is the grocery store?
Где находится продуктовый магазин?

Where is a telephone?
Где я могу найти телефон?

Where is the _____ Hotel?
Где гостиница _____?

Where may I buy batteries?
Где можно купить аккумуляторы?

I need some milk to drink.
Мне надо выпить молока.

I need to buy some insulin.
Мне надо купить инсулин.

I need to buy some insulin syringes.
Мне надо купить шприц для инсулина.

Japanese

Please help me. I have diabetes.
Watashi wa toonyoobyoo desu.
Tedasuke shite tadake nasu ka.

私 は 糖 尿 病 で す. 手 助 け し
て い た だ け ま す か.

May I please have some sugar or
fruit juice or Coke?
Satoo to jyuusu to koora wa
doko desu ka.

砂 糖 と ジ ュ ー ス と コ ー ラ は
何 処 で す か.

May I please have some milk?
Miruku o ne ga i shimasu.

ミ ル ク お 願 い し ま す.

My blood sugar is too low.
Watashi no ketochi wa totem tekui desu.

私 の 血 糖 値 は と て も て く い
で す.

I must have something to eat.
Ima nani ga taberu shitsuku go orimasu.

い ま な に が 食 べ る し つ く が
あ り ま す.

Where is the American Consulate?
Amerika no ryoojikan wa doko desu ka.

アメリカ の 大 使 館 は 何 処 で す か .

Where is the hospital?
Byooin wa doko desu ka.

病 院 は 何 処 で す か .

Where may I buy medicine?
Doko de kusuri ga kae masu ka.

何 処 で く す り が 買 え ま す か .

Where is the grocery store?
Suapoa maaketto wa doko desu ka.

ス ー パ は 何 処 で す か .

Where is the telephone?
Denwa wa doko desu ka.

電 話 は 何 処 で す か .

Where is the _____ Hotel?
_____ **hoteru wa doko desu ka.**

……… ホ テ ル は 何 処 で す か .

Where may I buy batteries?
Doko de denchi ga kaemasuka.

何 処 で 電 池 が 買 え ま す か .

I need to buy some insulin.
Doko de insulin ga kaemasuka.

何 処 で イ ン ス リ ン が 買 え ま
す か .

I need to buy some insulin syringes.
Doko de insulin chushia ga kaemasuka.

何 処 で イ ン ス リ ン 注 射 針 が 買
え ま す か .

Chinese

Please help me. I have diabetes.

請 幫 助 我. 我 有 糖 尿 病.

May I please have some sugar or
fruit juice or Coca Cola?

請 給 我 一 些 糖, 或 果 汁,
或 是 可 口 可 樂 好 嗎?

May I please have some milk?

請 給 我 一 些 牛 奶 好 嗎?

My blood sugar is too low.

我 的 血 糖 很 低.

I must have something to eat.

我 必 須 吃 點 東 西.

Where is the American Consulate?

請 問 美 國 領 事 館 在 那 裏?

Where is the hospital?

請 問 醫 院 在 那 裏?

Where may I buy medicine?

請 問 在 那 裏 可 以 買 藥 ?

Where is the grocery store?

請 問 超 市 在 那 裏?

Where is a telephone?

請 問 電 話 在 那 裏?

Where is the _____ Hotel?

請 問...... 旅 館 在 那 裏?

Where may I buy batteries?

請 問 在 那 裏 可 以 買 電 池?

I need to buy some insulin.

我 需 要 買 些 胰 島 素 製 劑.

I need to buy some insulin syringes.

我 需 要 買 些 胰 島 素 注 射 針.

Greek

I have diabetes.
Εψω ζαχαρο.
Eho zaharo.

I need sugar, orange juice, or a coca cola.
Θελω ζαχαρη, πορτοκαλαδα η ενα
γλυκο πιοτο.
The'lo zahaou, portokalada,
I ena coca cola.

Scuba Diving

Date:

To Whom It May Concern:

RE: (*Your name*)

Mr. _____ has diabetes and takes insulin. He has successfully completed a certified diving course. We have many patients who successfully scuba dive, and we recommend that:

1. The patient successfully completes a certified diving course.

2. The patient monitors his blood glucose before each dive. The blood glucose should be above 150 mg/dl before a dive. If it is less than 150 mg/dl, he should ingest 5 g of glucose for every 25 mg/dl under 150 mg/dl.

3. The patient should carry liquid or gel glucose during all dives.

4. The patient should follow the recommended dive tables.

5. The patient should dive with a companion who is able to treat low blood glucose (hypoglycemia).

6. The patient should not drink any alcohol for 24 hours before the time of the dive.

If you have any questions, please contact me.

Sincerely yours,

(*Provider's signature*)
Health care provider's name

Address _____

Telephone number _____

Index

About the American Diabetes Association

The American Diabetes Association is the nation's leading voluntary health organization supporting diabetes research, information, and advocacy. Its mission is to prevent and cure diabetes and to improve the lives of all people affected by diabetes. The American Diabetes Association is the leading publisher of comprehensive diabetes information. Its huge library of practical and authoritative books for people with diabetes covers every aspect of self-care—cooking and nutrition, fitness, weight control, medications, complications, emotional issues, and general self-care.

To order American Diabetes Association books: Call 1-800-232-6733. http://store.diabetes.org [Note: there is no need to use www when typing this particular Web address]

To join the American Diabetes Association: Call 1-800-806-7801. www.diabetes.org/membership

For more information about diabetes or ADA programs and services: Call 1-800-342-2383). E-mail: Customerservice@diabetes.org www.diabetes.org

To locate an ADA/NCQA Recognized Provider of quality diabetes care in your area: Call 1-703-549-1500 ext. 2202. www.diabetes.org/recognition/Physicians/ListAll.asp

To find an ADA Recognized Education Program in your area: Call 1-888-232-0822. www.diabetes.org/recognition/education.asp

To join the fight to increase funding for diabetes research, end discrimination, and improve insurance coverage: Call 1-800-342-2383. www.diabetes.org /advocacy

To find out how you can get involved with the programs in your community: Call 1-800-342-2383). See below for program Web addresses.

- *American Diabetes Month:* Educational activities aimed at those diagnosed with diabetes—month of November. www.diabetes.org/ADM
- *American Diabetes Alert:* Annual public awareness campaign to find the undiagnosed—held the fourth Tuesday in March. www.diabetes.org/alert
- *The Diabetes Assistance & Resources Program (DAR):* diabetes awareness program targeted to the Latino community. www.diabetes.org/DAR
- *African American Program:* diabetes awareness program targeted to the African American community. www.diabetes.org/africanamerican
- *Awakening the Spirit: Pathways to Diabetes Prevention & Control:* diabetes awareness program targeted to the Native American community. www.diabetes.org/awakening

To find out about an important research project regarding type 2 diabetes: www.diabetes.org/ada/research.asp

To obtain information on making a planned gift or charitable bequest: Call 1-888-700-7029. www.diabetes.org/ada/plan.asp

To make a donation or memorial contribution: Call 1-800-342-2383. www.diabetes.org/ada/cont.asp